Praise for

PCOS: THE DIETITIAN'S GUIDE

"A book that not only every practicing dietitian and nutritionist should have on their shelves, but any professional who comes into clinical contact with women suffering from PCOS. Women with PCOS will be well-armed to work with their doctors, dieticians, reproductive endocrinologists, and gynecologists to fight the symptoms of PCOS and its related issues."

— **Linda Harvey, Editor,** *PCOS Today Magazine*

"I just wanted to tell you that I think your book about PCOS is excellent! In addition to being a dietitian and a nurse, my 18 y/o daughter has PCOS. Your book includes the best explanation of the physiology as well as evidence-based nutrition information on the topic. I am grateful for the information for personal reasons and also for the opportunity for the CEUs."

— **Jackie Monahan, RN, RD**

"This book fills a gap in the practical literature on medical nutrition therapy for Polycystic Ovary Syndrome. It is a useful, practice-oriented book written by an experienced dietitian for dietitians. I highly recommend this book for dietitians interested in women's health."

— **Jeffrey E. Harris, DrPH, MPH, RD, LDN**

"Dietitians really need to be the leaders in the management of PCOS and your book is a step in the right direction."

— **Judy Simon MS,RD,CDE**

"Thank you for creating such a well-researched resource! I feel much better equipped to treat my patients with PCOS and suspected PCOS patients now."

— **Leslie Lawton, RD, CDE**

"This is a very important book, and it is written very clearly and professionally. I will share it with my colleagues in Israel."

— **Ilana Dariel, RD, PhD**

"A great resource for the women who truly need an expert to help them with this difficult and too little studied syndrome. Thank you for your gift to the world!"

— **Mary Farkas, M.S., M.A.**

PCOS
THE DIETITIAN'S GUIDE

Angela Grassi, MS, RD, LDN

Luca Publishing
551 West Lancaster Avenue
Suite 305
Haverford, PA 19041
(484) 252-9028
www.PCOSnutrition.com

PCOS: The Dietitian's Guide, 2nd edition
Written by Angela Grassi

This is a completely revised edition of The Dietitian's Guide to Polycystic
Ovary Syndrome, published in North America by Luca Publishing in 2007.

Cataloging-in-Publication Data is available
from the U.S. Library of Congress.
ISBN: 978-0-9851164-2-2

Edited by Tracy Denninger
tracymdenn@gmail.com

Interior design by Emily Avedissian
www.emilyavedissian.com

Cover design by Peri Poloni-Gabriel, Knockout Design
www.knocloutbooks.com

Manufactured in the United States of America

TABLE OF CONTENTS

REVIEWERS

ACKNOWLEDGEMENTS

Writing the 2ⁿᵈ edition of this book was a journey that took one year to complete. Along the way, I experienced many obstacles and life challenges including the death of my father who taught me determination and that anything was possible if you set your mind to it. There were joyful times too: weddings, the birth of my niece Molly, and many toddler and Kindergarten milestones. I have many people to thank for their support and contribution in the completion of this book and for keeping me on this journey.

First, I want to thank Emily Avedissian for her hard work and talent on the interior design of this book.

Thank you to Peri Poloni-Gabriel for designing such a fantastic cover. I have such admiration for your talent.

Thank you Tracy Denninger for all your hard work editing this 2ⁿᵈ edition. You did a fantastic job getting this book ready for print.

Thank you Lisa Marasco for sharing your insightful and well-written thesis showing the connection between PCOS and insufficient milk supply.

Thank you to Jessica Setnick, my soul-sister dietitian, for reviewing this book and for your support, encouragement, and friendship.

To my good friend, Dr. Stephanie Mattei: you are a lifesaver and I cannot thank you enough. Thank you for co-authoring Psychological Aspects of PCOS and for reviewing this book. You are such an awesome mom and therapist. I appreciate your time, expertise, support, and friendship.

Thank you also to Michelle Shwarz for co-authoring the chapter on Psychological Aspects of PCOS and for being so dedicated to supporting women with PCOS.

To Dr. Katherine Sherif, I can't express how much admiration and respect I have for you as a friend and physician. Your kindness, compassion, and expertise are exactly what women with PCOS need. Thank you for writing the chapter on Understanding PCOS. The book would not be complete without it.

Natalie Ritchey, thank you for your creative menu contributions. You have a bright future ahead!

Thank you to Amy Ogle for reviewing the chapter Pregnancy, Lactation, and the Postpartum Period. I appreciate your time and expertise.

Judy Simon, thank you for contributing your intriguing case study and for your dedication to PCOS and helping women become moms.

I want to thank Dr. Jeff Harris for editing the first edition of this book. I cannot thank you enough for your endless support, expertise, respect, and encouragement. Never have I met a professor liked so much by both his students and colleagues.

Patricia Davidson, you were just what we needed at the final hour. Thank you for all your hard work and time in co-authoring such a comprehensive chapter, Nutritional Strategies and Lifestyle Modification for PCOS.

A heart felt special thank you to Dr. Lynn Monahan Couch who I truly believe, is a gift sent to me from God. Thank you Lynn for all of your hard work, time, and dedication in editing and reviewing this book, for co-authoring the chapter Nutritional Strategies and Lifestyle Modifications for PCOS, for contributing a case study and most of all, for your friendship. I greatly appreciate all your effort, advice, and encouragement. It has been wonderful working with you and forming the friendship we have. I applaud your enthusiasm and passion for PCOS. This book wouldn't be complete without you.

Lastly, I would also like to thank my family and friends for all their love and support. Most of all, thank you to the men in my life. Luca and Henry, who bring me such joy and remind me that there is more in life than PCOS. And of course to Chris, my biggest fan and special gift from God, I am so blessed to have you in my life. I could not have done this without your endless love, support and kindness. I love you so much.

INTRODUCTION

I felt compelled to write this book, first published in 2007 as *The Dietitian's Guide to Polycystic Ovary Syndrome*, for several reasons. The first is that PCOS the most complex endocrine disorder among women of reproductive age and there has been much confusion surrounding its diagnosis and treatment approaches among the medical community. This has led to numerous misdiagnoses and immense frustration and anger in women who have PCOS, all of which could have been avoided with adequate knowledge of the syndrome. Furthermore, women with PCOS are at an increased risk for obesity, cardiovascular disease, diabetes, cancer, depression, infertility, and miscarriage; early intervention aimed at preventing these is crucial.

Current treatment recommendations for PCOS emphasize the importance of dietary and lifestyle modification, thus increasing the number of referrals to dietitians for nutrition management. However, many dietitians may lack the knowledge and training to recognize or effectively treat individuals with PCOS. Some dietitians have never even heard of PCOS before. This may result from the lack of clinical studies regarding diet composition and PCOS, or because the syndrome was viewed primarily as a reproductive disorder and not diagnosed as readily as it is today. Personally, I had never heard of PCOS until after I had graduated with my master's degree in nutrition and was already working as a dietitian for a year.

Another reason I wanted to write this book is because I have PCOS and like too many women, I was misdiagnosed until I was in my late 20's. In fact, when I was diagnosed with PCOS I was already familiar with the syndrome. As a dietitian, I had treated numerous women with PCOS, yet was unable to fully recognize it for myself. This led me to question: if I hadn't been able to recognize PCOS for myself when I was already familiar with it, how are other dietitians, health professionals, or even patients going to be able to recognize it?

I remember the first time I had ever heard of PCOS. It was in the year 2000 and I was working as an outpatient nutritionist for an eating disorder treatment facility. Sally, my patient who had bulimia nervosa, was recently diagnosed with PCOS when I met her. Never hearing of PCOS before, I immediately began researching the syndrome only to find limited information. The information that did exist described PCOS as a reproductive disorder associated with elevated insulin and androgen levels, weight gain, and obesity. A very low carbohydrate diet was recommended.

It was at that time when I first questioned whether I had PCOS. Since puberty I have been overweight even though I have always been physically active. I never had any of the classic PCOS symptoms of excess hair growth, acne, or irregular periods, therefore, I didn't think it was possible that I could have PCOS (and I was told this by numerous physicians).

After my encounter with that first patient, I started to see many other patients like her. It was also at this time that I started gaining weight out of the blue-and it was all accumulating in my mid-section. I attributed the weight gain (2-3 pounds per month) to many factors: a sedentary job, decreased metabolism, birth control pills, more eating and less physical activity. Being a dietitian, I started writing down and analyzing everything that I ate. I was not eating any more than I had before and I was certainly not eating enough to produce the weight gain that I was experiencing. It didn't make sense.

I went to see my internist to get blood work done. I suggested the possibility of having PCOS. She said, however, that she could not test for it because I was on birth control pills and they would affect the results of my hormone levels. She also said that since I always had regular periods, I could not have PCOS. All my lab results came back normal. Her answer to me about the weight gain was "watch your diet." So I figured, as I had for most of my life, that my weight was my fault.

I started noticing some other things that weren't right. For instance, I craved carbohydrates, especially sweets, and I sometimes experienced hypoglycemic episodes. My first encounter with hypoglycemia was in my senior year of college when I woke up one morning dizzy and nauseous. After eating breakfast, I got extremely dizzy to the point where I could not walk straight and had to stop and rest. I went to the health center where they diagnosed me with vertigo, said I had a virus that was going around, and prescribed me antivert. The next day I got a call telling me that the results of blood work showed my glucose reading was 40 mg/dl (normal is 70-99).

I had always wondered why I experienced hypoglycemia that day and days since. I was careful, eating frequently and including sufficient protein with my meals and snacks. My fasting blood glucose levels had always been normal, yet I would still experience hypoglycemia at times. Several months after seeing my internist, I wasn't experiencing any change in my weight and decided to see another physician.

This time, not only did I suggest PCOS to my doctor but asked to get an oral glucose tolerance test done in addition to more lab tests. When the doctor called me with the results, she said all my hormone levels were fine and that the oral glucose tolerance test showed I had hypoglycemia (I already knew that!). She suggested I follow the South Beach Diet to lose weight and manage my hypoglycemia. What I didn't realize at the time was that she never checked my fasting insulin with the glucose test. She only tested my glucose and was not thorough in checking the hormones needed to diagnose PCOS. It also appeared that my triglyceride levels, still in normal range, were much higher than they had been the last time I had them done. I decided to stop taking birth control medication to see if my weight and triglycerides would decrease. My weight did not change and I still experienced regular periods.

A year later, my husband and I were starting to think about starting a family. At the same time, Dr. Katherine Sherif, a well-known physician who specializes in PCOS and women's health, moved back to the Philadelphia area. I made an appointment to see her and knew that if I had PCOS, she would be the one to tell me. I had to know once and for all if I had PCOS or not, especially before trying to conceive a child.

Dr. Sherif was a model for what we wish all doctors would be: kind, compassionate, brilliant, and thorough. She took a detailed medical history on me and agreed that I should be able to lose weight with all the exercise I was doing and for the amount that I was eating. I finally felt validated that it was not my fault I wasn't able to lose weight. She also examined my skin and immediately noticed signs of acanthosis nigricans (markers of elevated insulin) on the back of my neck and knuckles. Since I am fair skinned, it had been difficult to see them. Dr. Sherif agreed that I did not have the typical symptoms of PCOS and that I would have to get an ultrasound done and comprehensive blood work to rule out any other possible medical conditions. Later that week, I went for an ultrasound. I immediately saw the classic string of pearls around my ovaries and it was then that I knew my instincts were correct: I had PCOS.

My blood work came back with elevated insulin and luteinizing hormone, and androgen levels so high that Dr. Sherif, who is Middle Eastern, remarked that if she had my levels she would probably have a full beard. I started taking Metformin and soon started experiencing fewer cravings for carbohydrates. I cut back slightly on my carbohydrate intake and made sure the grains I was eating were always whole and unprocessed as possible. Although my weight did not change much, after a year of treatment with Metformin and changes in my diet, I was able to get my insulin levels into normal ranges and my lipid panel had greatly improved. My husband and I conceived our first child, a son, with no difficulty one year after I was diagnosed with PCOS and started treatment. Three years later, we conceived our second son, also without difficulty. I did not experience any medical complications with either pregnancies and both babies were full-term and healthy.

Although my symptoms weren't typical, my instinct that I had PCOS was strong, driving my search for answers. Today, nearly a decade after my diagnosis, my search for answers and evidence-based nutrition information for PCOS continues. So much more is known about PCOS since the first edition of this book was published over six years ago. PCOS is now viewed as primarily an endocrine disorder with metabolic consequences that continue past menopause. At least 10 different phenotypes of PCOS have been identified, requiring research going forward to specify phenotype using the agreed upon Rotterdam criteria. While the optimal diet composition remains unclear, the role of diet and lifestyle in managing PCOS is more evident than ever. Like the majority of people, women with PCOS turn to the internet for nutrition information. Unfortunately, not all the nutrition information for PCOS is evidence-based. In fact, some advice may cause women more harm than good. This book is written to give you, the dietitian, the knowledge and training needed to recognize PCOS among your clients (or even yourselves). It is my hope that you use this knowledge to provide effective, evidenced-based medical nutrition therapy to help women improve their symptoms, become mothers, prevent further medical complications, and live healthier lives.

Angela Grassi, MS, RD, LDN

For Chris and Frank

Chapter 1

UNDERSTANDING PCOS

By Katherine D. Sherif, MD, FACP

WHAT IS PCOS?

Polycystic ovary syndrome (PCOS) is a complex genetic disorder of androgen excess, ovulatory dysfunction, and polycystic ovaries.[1] Worldwide, PCOS affects 6% to 10% of women,[2-5] making it the most common endocrinopathy in women of reproductive age.

First recognized in 1935 by gynecologists Irving F. Stein and Michael L. Leventhol for its relationship to menstrual disturbances, PCOS is associated with a collection of reproductive abnormalities: polycystic ovaries, menstrual irregularity, infertility, and hyperandrogenism. However, the majority of women diagnosed with PCOS have abnormal metabolic parameters such as insulin resistance, central obesity, and dyslipidemia.

With time and more understanding of this complex disease, PCOS is no longer considered solely a reproductive disorder but also an endocrine disorder. In December 2012, the National Institutes of Health (NIH) held an evidence-based methodology workshop on PCOS, during which the recommendation was made to change the name of the condition now known as PCOS to "one that reflects the complex metabolic, hypothalamic, pituitary, ovarian, and adrenal interactions that characterize the syndrome."[6]

The etiology of PCOS is unknown, but a genetic link has been identified. Many women with PCOS have female relatives on either the maternal or paternal side with a history of irregular periods and/or infertility. PCOS appears to be polygenic, with multiple types of gene mutations seeming to cause similar symptoms.

In the past, an abnormal hypothalamic-pituitary-ovarian axis was identified as the basic etiology. However, it has become more clear that the hormone insulin plays a central role in the pathophysiology. Lifestyle and environmental factors strongly influence the expression of PCOS, with weight gain worsening both the metabolic and reproductive parameters.[1] Approximately 40% to 74% of women with PCOS are obese.[3,7] However, even lean and normal-weight women with PCOS can have hyperinsulinemia and insulin resistance.[8]

PATHOPHYSIOLOGY OF PCOS

Figure 1 shows the pathophysiology of PCOS. As part of the condition, there is increased ovarian production of androgens, both androstenedione and testosterone. The increased androgens may be due to insulin.[9] There are insulin receptors on the theca cells of the uterus. Increased insulin stimulates the uterine theca cells to increase the production of androstenedione and testosterone,[10] which inhibits ovulation and causes androgenic symptoms. Insulin also reduces the sex hormone-binding globulin (SHBG), which binds to testosterone, resulting in greater amounts of free testosterone and affecting follicular development.[11]

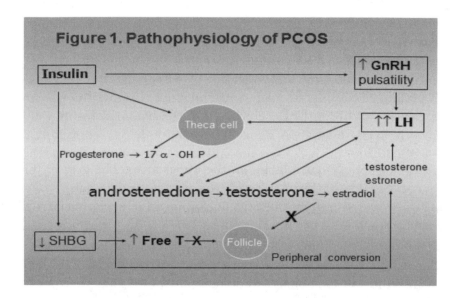

Figure 1. Pathophysiology of PCOS

Increased androgens also may be the result of increased gonadotropin releasing-hormone (GnRH) pulsatility.[12] Rapid, high-amplitude pulses increase luteinizing hormone (LH) secretion preferentially over follicle-stimulating hormone (FSH). Elevated LH stimulates androgen production from the theca cells, and androstenedione that is converted to estrone in the periphery stimulates more LH secretion. Although hyperinsulinemia results from insulin resistance, it is unknown why GnRH has increased pulsatility in women with PCOS favoring the increase in LH.

In women with PCOS compared with those without the condition, serum LH responses following GnRH are exaggerated. In addition to driving the release of LH, GnRH primes the pituitary gland to enhance subsequent responses to GnRH stimulation, so there is profoundly increased gonatrophic sensitivity to GnRH in PCOS. To complicate matters, testosterone inhibits the negative feedback of estradiol and progesterone on GnRH, so LH continues to be released. Additionally, insulin significantly amplifies LH responses to GnRH.

PCOS symptoms can be attributed to two underlying processes: hyperinsulinemia and hyperandrogenemia. Hyperinsulinemia is associated with weight gain, which causes insulin resistance and subsequent hyperinsulinemia, which in turn causes weight gain. The vicious cycle of insulin resistance favors weight gain despite good nutrition and exercise.

Hyperinsulinemia causes acanthosis nigricans, which is Latin for "black skin." In people with dark skin, acanthosis nigricans is easily detected as dark, soft skin on the back of the neck and on the elbows, knees, and underarms; between the breasts; and across the knuckles and groin. For people with lighter skin, it may manifest as skin that appears tan above the neckline and rough grey elbows. Hyperinsulinemia also causes skin tags and follicular keratosis, or reddened rough hair follicles on the upper arms. The greater the hyperinsulinemia, the more severe the acanthosis nigricans.

The other symptoms of PCOS, including an irregular menstrual cycle and infertility, are caused by high androgens, primarily testosterone, produced by the ovaries. Other androgenic symptoms include severe acne and hirsutism of the face, chest, back, lower abdomen, or upper shoulders. One of the most distressing PCOS symptoms that women report is androgenic alopecia, or diffuse loss of scalp hair.

CONDITIONS ASSOCIATED WITH PCOS

The United States spends an estimated $4 billion annually to identify and manage PCOS,[6] representing a major health and economic burden. As shown in Table 1.1, women with PCOS have been found to have an increased prevalence of multiple cardiovascular risk factors. Dyslipidemia may be the most common metabolic abnormality as low high-density lipoprotein (HDL) cholesterol levels and high triglyceride (TG) levels are commonly found in women with PCOS.[13]

Insulin resistance occurs in approximately 50% to 70% of women with PCOS and in 95% of obese women with the syndrome.[14] Both lean and obese women with PCOS have a greater waist circumference than women without PCOS.[15] Excess upper body fat is associated with insulin resistance.[16] Insulin has been shown to be a risk factor for type 2 diabetes (T2DM) in women with PCOS, independent of weight.[17,18] Furthermore, PCOS is associated with a 2.5-fold increased prevalence of impaired glucose tolerance and a fourfold increased prevalence of T2DM.[19] The International Diabetes Federation recognizes PCOS as a nonmodifiable risk factor for T2DM.[20] Additionally, women with PCOS are at an increased risk of metabolic syndrome compared with age-matched healthy women without PCOS. [21,22]

Table 1.1: Prevalence of Cardiovascular Disease Risk Factors in PCOS

CVD Risk Factor	% of women with PCOS
Abnormal glucose metabolism	50 to 70[19]
Dyslipidemia	70[23]
Obesity	40 to 74[3,7]
Insulin resistance	50 to 80[14,19]
Metabolic syndrome	24 to 47[21,22,24]

PCOS is associated with many other adverse health risks (see Table 1.2), including an increased risk of endometrial cancer, which may result from irregular bleeding or amenorrhea, and an increased risk of nonalcoholic fatty liver disease (NAFLD), which worsens in response to increases in adipose tissue and insulin resistance.[25] Another associated health risk is obstructive sleep apnea, which results not only from obesity but also from elevated androgens that cause apnea through a central brain mechanism. Women with PCOS are also at an increased risk of venous thromboembolism.[26]

Anxiety and depression are common in PCOS and can compound overweight by causing a lack of motivation to eat well and exercise. Women with PCOS are more likely to develop hypothyroidism,[27,28] which is associated with fatigue, depression, infertility, weight gain, and alopecia. Women with PCOS also have a higher incidence of gestational diabetes, miscarriages, preterm deliveries, and still-births,[29] but it is not clear whether these problems stem from high androgen or insulin levels.

Table 1.2: Other Conditions Associated with PCOS

- Endometrial cancer
- Hypothyroidism
- Coagulpathy
- Autoimmune disorders
- Obstructive sleep apnea
- Eating disorders
- NAFLD
- Mood disorders (anxiety and depression)

DIAGNOSIS

In the past, the absence of definitive criteria for PCOS have made it difficult to diagnose and especially difficult to compare studies. Table 1.3 shows the three different diagnostic criteria.

In 1990, the NIH recommended that the criteria for diagnosing PCOS include hyperandrogenism and/or hyperandrogenemia, oligo-ovulation, and the exclusion of other known disorders. In 2003, the European Society for Human Reproduction and the American Society for Reproductive Medicine met in Rotterdam and expanded the NIH criteria to include a presentation of two of the following three criteria: oligo- and/or anovulation, hyperandrogenemic symptoms and/or elevated serum androgens, and polycystic ovaries confirmed by transvaginal ultrasound. The expanded Rotterdam criteria include all women with PCOS as defined by the 1990 NIH criteria but also women with either clinical and/or biochemical hyperandrogenism and polycystic ovaries.

In 2006, the Androgen Excess PCOS Society (AEPCOS) recommended that PCOS be defined by clinical and/or biochemical hyperandrogenism and oligoanovulation and/or polycystic ovaries, excluding other endocrinopathies and supporting the NIH criteria.[30] The AEPCOS emphasized that PCOS should first be considered a disorder of androgen excess or hyperandrogenism[30] and takes into account that not all women with PCOS have polycystic ovaries or experience oligoanovulation.

Table 1.3: Diagnostic Criteria for PCOS

NIH (1990)	Rotterdam (2003)	AEPCOS Society (2006)
• Chronic anovulation • Clinical and/or biochemical signs of hyperandrogenism (with exclusion of other etiologies, e.g., congenital adrenal hyperplasia) (Both criteria needed)	• Oligo- and/or anovulation • Clinical and/or biochemical signs of hyperandrogenism • Polycystic ovaries (Two of three criteria needed)	• Clinical and/or biochemical signs of hyperandrogenism • Ovarian dysfunction (oligoanovulation and/or polycystic ovarian morphology) (Both criteria needed)

After reviewing the benefits and drawbacks of the different diagnostic criteria, the final report from the NIH Evidenced-based Methodology Workshop on PCOS held in 2012 recommends maintaining the Rotterdam criteria (which include the NIH and AEPCOS criteria)[6]:

- androgen excess + ovulatory dysfunction
- androgen excess + polycystic ovarian morphology
- ovulatory dysfunction + polycystic ovarian morphology
- androgen excess + ovulatory dysfunction + polycystic ovarian morphology

The NIH Workshop recommended that specific phenotypes be reported in all research studies, clinical care, professional journals, funding sources, and professional societies.[6]

PATIENT HEALTH HISTORY

As a practitioner who diagnoses and treats girls and women with PCOS, there are clinical manifestations, patterns of symptoms during puberty, and treatment plans that are effective in normalizing PCOS parameters.

A patient's history is the most important element in diagnosing PCOS, followed by a physical examination and blood tests. The typical history reveals menarche, on average, at 12 to 13 years old. Almost immediately, menses occur at irregular intervals. Often teenagers will be told that irregular menses are a normal part of development and that they will "grow out of it."

At this point, girls are often prescribed oral contraceptive pills (OCPs) to initiate regular menses prior to the establishment of a PCOS diagnosis. OCPs result in lower serum androgen levels, decreased ovarian androgen production, and improvements in menstrual cyclicity, hirsutism, and acne and, in fact, form a mainstay of therapy. However, OCPs may delay diagnosis because a patient may now report regular menses.

After a period of some years, these women often discontinue OCPs, perhaps to conceive, and resume a pattern of irregular menses. At this point, they often turn to a gynecologist, perhaps blaming OCPs for their menstrual irregularity and infertility rather than addressing the underlying condition that led to the need for hormonal contraception in the first place.

PHYSICAL EXAMINATION

The most important component for diagnosing PCOS is the physical examination. Elevated blood pressure (in the 130s/80s) may be found when taking vital signs. Most women with PCOS have central obesity consisting of visceral fat deposition in the abdomen, upper arms, and upper back. Therefore, PCOS may be overlooked in women who are slender.

Hirsutism may be present on the face, neck, chest, periareolar area, upper arms, back, or abdomen. Even just a few terminal hairs on the chest, between the breasts, or on the lower abdomen indicate elevated serum androgens. Acne can range from nonexistent to severe and be present anywhere on the body. Diffuse alopecia also is common.

It is important to remember that not all women with PCOS have all the symptoms listed above. The phenotypic presentations vary because the etiology is multifactorial. For example, some women may not have the testosterone receptors in skin that cause hirsutism, especially women of East Asian descent. Other women may have a normal body mass index (BMI) and still have PCOS. Some women do not have acne or alopecia. A very small number will have regular menses but most of the other features of hyperandrogenism and polycystic ovaries. Therefore, the absence of all classically described symptoms should not automatically exclude PCOS.

LABORATORY VALUES

It is important to note that blood values obtained while a patient is on OCPs are not useful in diagnosing PCOS. Patients should be off OCPs for at least six weeks before measuring hormone levels. A list of lab tests used to diagnose and monitor PCOS can be found in Table 1.4.

The most useful lab test in a PCOS workup is total testosterone. Total testosterone greater than 50 ng/dL is considered elevated; free testosterone is a less reliable measurement.[30] Other confirmatory labs include a LH-to-FSH ratio of greater than 2.

Serum insulin measurements can help determine the presence of insulin resistance. An insulin level below 10 is considered normal. However, a blood specimen used to analyze serum insulin must be frozen quickly and, in a typical office setting, this may not happen. Also, it may be allowed to thaw on the way to the lab. Either scenario results in erroneously low insulin levels.

There is a rapid progression from impaired glucose tolerance (IGT) to T2DM in women with PCOS.[31] For this reason, the AEPCOS recommends screening for T2DM with a two-hour oral glucose tolerance test (OGTT) every two years in women with PCOS who have normal glucose levels and annually in those with elevated glucose levels.[31]

Other conditions that can cause irregular menstrual cycles must be ruled out before diagnosing PCOS. All women with a history of

Table 1.4: Laboratory Tests to Diagnose and Monitor PCOS

Lab Test	Result
Free testosterone	Elevated
Total testosterone	Elevated
LH-to-FSH ratio	Elevated
DHEA sulfate	Elevated
Fasting glucose	Elevated
Fasting insulin	Elevated
TSH and thyroid peroxidase antibodies	Elevated
CRP	Elevated
Lipid profile	Elevated
HDL cholesterol	Decreased
Liver function tests	Elevated
OGTT	Elevated

irregular menses should have the following initial tests: pregnancy, prolactin level (to rule out a prolactin-secreting pituitary adenoma), and thyroid-stimulating hormone (TSH) (to rule out hypo- or hyperthyroidism). Other tests, which follow, can be performed depending on the clinical presentation:

- Cushing's disease in a patient with moon fascies, buffalo hump, central obesity and abdominal striae, and very thin arms and legs in relation to obesity. Check 24-hour urine for cortisol.
- Androgen-secreting tumor in a patient with sudden virilizing symptoms. Check DHEA sulfate (not DHEA).
- Late-onset (or nonclassical) congenital adrenal hyperplasia in a woman of Greek, Jewish, Latino, or Italian descent with precocious puberty. Check DNA test for common mutations of the 21-hydroxylase gene.

A fasting lipid profile is useful for assessing cardiovascular risk along with C-reactive protein (CRP) levels, which have been shown to be higher in women with PCOS.[31] After treatment begins, it is helpful to repeat blood tests in three to six months to assess the change in testosterone and improvement in lipid profile.

Transvaginal Sonography

Transvaginal sonography is necessary for infertility evaluation and management. However, if a patient does not wish to conceive and if she has a classic history and signs of PCOS, a transvaginal ultrasound without evidence of polycystic ovaries probably would not change management. The classic PCOS finding on a transvaginal ultrasound is a string of pearls, which describes typical cysts on at least one ovary that are peripheral, multiple, and less than 10 mm in diameter.

Despite the name polycystic ovary syndrome, 10% to 30% of women with PCOS do not show cysts on their ovaries.[32] The cysts result from hormonal imbalances rather than cause them.

MEDICAL TREATMENT OF PCOS

The goals of treatment for PCOS are to decrease symptoms, improve fertility, and prevent lifelong health risks. Lifestyle change should be the first approach to managing PCOS,[33] with medical treatment used in conjunction with lifestyle change.

In overweight women with PCOS, weight loss improves both metabolic and reproductive parameters. Medications include hormonal contraception, androgen blockers, and insulin sensitizers. Physician visits should be about every three months to evaluate the effect of medications, especially at the beginning of treatment.

The most commonly used medication for treatment of PCOS is OCPs. The supraphysiologic doses of estrogen suppress FSH and LH and induce regular periods. Estrogen also increases SHBG in the liver, which binds free testosterone and makes it unavailable to tissues. Acne may improve dramatically, and hirsutism and alopecia often decrease with OCP use. However, OCPs may negatively impact metabolic parameters, including CRP, TG, and insulin resistance.[34,35]

Spironolactone is a weak antihypertensive medication that effectively treats hirsutism and alopecia, and may be used alone or in combination with other medications. An androgen blocker, spironolactone competes with testosterone for androgen receptors. Although it may take three to six months to see an effect, the improvement in alopecia can be striking. Because spironolactone does not dramatically lower blood pressure, patients rarely, if ever, experience hypotension. However, this drug is a potent teratogen and must not be used in women who may become pregnant.

Metformin, an insulin sensitizer, can help patients surmount hyperinsulinemia, especially in conjunction with a healthy diet and exercise.[36] Through its effect on lowering insulin levels, metformin aids weight loss, decreases testosterone levels, induces ovulation, improves lipid profile, and lowers blood pressure.[34,37,38] The drug works by suppressing gluconeogenesis, increasing liver and muscle cells' sensitivity to insulin, and decreasing carbohydrate absorption.[38] Metformin can safely be taken during pregnancy and has even been shown to decrease first-trimester miscarriages that are common in PCOS.[34]

Since metformin is commonly associated with gastrointestinal (GI) effects such as nausea, bloating, and diarrhea, it should be titrated slowly and taken after meals. The extended-release form may minimize GI side effects and be better tolerated. The average dose of metformin for women with PCOS is 1,500 to 2,000 mg daily.

Women should be reminded that metformin is so effective in inducing ovulation that if they do not want to conceive, they must use contraception, even if they never have before.

Byetta, Victoza, and Bydureon are part of the newer class of injectable insulin sensitizers called GLP-1 receptor agonists, which share similar glucoregulatory properties as the hormone glucagon-like peptide-1 (GLP-1). GLP-1 receptor agonists may help women with PCOS improve insulin sensitivity and lose weight when metformin alone isn't effective. GLP-1 receptor agonists also are associated with GI side effects such as nausea, vomiting, and diarrhea, so dose titration can reduce these effects as with metformin.

Thiazolidinediones, mainly Actos and Avandia, are another class of insulin-sensitizing drugs previously used for PCOS treatment. However, these drugs have been found to have significant side effects, including weight gain and edema. Additionally, Avandia was shown to increase the risk of coronary heart disease (CHD) and heart attacks, while Actos has been linked to bladder cancer.[39] Subsequently, these medications are no longer recommended to treat women with PCOS.

Ovarian drilling is an old method of surgically reducing the size of the ovaries, which are enlarged in PCOS. By decreasing ovarian mass, fewer androgens are produced. Although ovarian drilling can be effective in improving PCOS symptoms, it is no longer considered the treatment of choice.

In summary, PCOS, a leading cause of menstrual irregularities and infertility, is also associated with obesity, hirsutism, and cardiovascular risk factors such as hyperlipidemia and impaired glucose tolerance. Diagnosis is based on a patient's history of menstrual dysfunction and evidence of hyperandrogenemia. Insulin resistance appears to play a central role in the pathophysiology.

Treatment is comprised of physical activity, proper nutrition, and weight loss. OCPs induce monthly menstrual cycles and improve acne and hirsutism. Insulin sensitizers such as metformin induce ovulation and improve metabolic parameters.

Research should focus on understanding the etiology of the severe insulin resistance seen in PCOS phenotypes as well as genetic causes, improved methods and criteria to assess PCOS, and optimal therapies to treat PCOS and achieve successful pregnancy.

REFERENCES

1. Goodarzi MO, Dumesic DA, Chazenbalk G, Azziz R. Polycystic ovary syndrome: etiology, pathogenesis and diagnosis. Nature reviews. Endocrinology. 2011;7(4):219-231.

2. Asuncion M, Calvo RM, San Millan JL, Sancho J, Avila S, Escobar-Morreale HF. A prospective study of the prevalence of the polycystic ovary syndrome in unselected Caucasian women from Spain. J Clin Endocrinol Metab. 2000;85(7):2434-2438.

3. Azziz R, Woods KS, Reyna R, Key TJ, Knochenhauer ES, Yildiz BO. The prevalence and features of the polycystic ovary syndrome in an unselected population. J Clin Endocrinol Metab. 2004;89(6):2745-2749.

4. Diamanti-Kandarakis E, Kouli CR, Bergiele AT, et al. A survey of the polycystic ovary syndrome in the Greek island of Lesbos: hormonal and metabolic profile. J Clin Endocrinol Metab. 1999;84(11):4006-4011.

5. Knochenhauer ES, Key TJ, Kahsar-Miller M, Waggoner W, Boots LR, Azziz R. Prevalence of the polycystic ovary syndrome in unselected black and white women of the southeastern United States: a prospective study. J Clin Endocrinol Metab. 1998;83(9):3078-3082.

6. Evidenced-based Methodology Workshop Executive Summary. Washington D.C.: National Institutes of Health; December 2012.

7. Yildiz BO, Knochenhauer ES, Azziz R. Impact of obesity on the risk for polycystic ovary syndrome. J Clin Endocrinol Metab. 2008;93(1):162-168.

8. Wang ET, Calderon-Margalit R, Cedars MI, et al. Polycystic ovary syndrome and risk for long-term diabetes and dyslipidemia. Obstetrics and gynecology. 2011;117(1):6-13.

9. Dunaif A. Insulin resistance and the polycystic ovary syndrome: mechanism and implications for pathogenesis. Endocrine reviews. 1997;18(6):774-800.

10. Nelson VL, Legro RS, Strauss JF, 3rd, McAllister JM. Augmented androgen production is a stable steroidogenic phenotype of propagated theca cells from polycystic ovaries. Molecular endocrinology (Baltimore, Md.). 1999;13(6):946-957.

11. Sherif K, Kushner H, Falkner BE. Sex hormone-binding globulin and insulin resistance in African-American women. Metabolism. 1998;47(1):70-74.

12. Rebar R, Judd HL, Yen SS, Rakoff J, Vandenberg G, Naftolin F. Characterization of the inappropriate gonadotropin secretion in polycystic ovary syndrome. J Clin Invest. 1976;57(5):1320-1329.

13. Sharma ST, Nestler JE. Prevention of diabetes and cardiovascular disease in women with PCOS: treatment with insulin sensitizers. Best Pract Res Clin Endocrinol Metab. 2006;20(2):245-260.

14. DeUgarte CM, Bartolucci AA, Azziz R. Prevalence of insulin resistance in the polycystic ovary syndrome using the homeostasis model assessment. Fertil Steril. 2005;83(5):1454-1460.

15. Cascella T, Palomba S, De Sio I, et al. Visceral fat is associated with cardiovascular risk in women with polycystic ovary syndrome. Hum Reprod. 2008;23(1):153-159.

16. Garruti G, Depalo R, Vita MG, et al. Adipose tissue, metabolic syndrome and polycystic ovary syndrome: from pathophysiology to treatment. Reproductive biomedicine online. 2009;19(4):552-563.

17. Corbould A. Insulin resistance in skeletal muscle and adipose tissue in polycystic ovary syndrome: are the molecular mechanisms distinct from type 2 diabetes? Panminerva medica. 2008;50(4):279-294.

18. Dunaif A, Segal KR, Futterweit W, Dobrjansky A. Profound peripheral insulin resistance, independent of obesity, in polycystic ovary syndrome. Diabetes. 1989;38(9):1165-1174.

19. Moran LJ, Misso ML, Wild RA, Norman RJ. Impaired glucose tolerance, type 2 diabetes and metabolic syndrome in polycystic ovary syndrome: a systematic review and meta-analysis. Human Repro Update. 2010;16(4):347-363.

20. Alberti KG, Zimmet P, Shaw J. International Diabetes Federation: a consensus on Type 2 diabetes prevention. Diabetic Med. 2007;24(5):451-463.

21. Dokras A, Bochner M, Hollinrake E, Markham S, Vanvoorhis B, Jagasia DH. Screening women with polycystic ovary syndrome for metabolic syndrome. Obstetrics and gynecology. 2005;106(1):131-137.

22. Ehrmann DA, Liljenquist DR, Kasza K, Azziz R, Legro RS, Ghazzi MN. Prevalence and predictors of the metabolic syndrome in women with polycystic ovary syndrome. J Clin Endocrinol Metab. 2006;91(1):48-53.

23. Legro RS, Kunselman AR, Dunaif A. Prevalence and predictors of dyslipidemia in women with polycystic ovary syndrome. Amer journal med. 2001;111(8):607-613.

24. Hudecova M, Holte J, Olovsson M, Larsson A, Berne C, Sundstrom-Poromaa I. Prevalence of the metabolic syndrome in women with a previous diagnosis of polycystic ovary syndrome: long-term follow-up. Fertil steril. 2011;96(5):1271-1274.

25. Baranova A, Tran TP, Birerdinc A, Younossi ZM. Systematic review: association of polycystic ovary syndrome with metabolic syndrome and non-alcoholic

fatty liver disease. Aliment pharmacol ther. 2011;33(7):801-814.

26. Bird ST, Hartzema AG, Brophy JM, Etminan M, Delaney JA. Risk of venous thromboembolism in women with polycystic ovary syndrome: a population-based matched cohort analysis. CMAJ. 2013;185(2):E115-120.

27. Kachuei M, Jafari F, Kachuei A, Keshteli AH. Prevalence of autoimmune thyroiditis in patients with polycystic ovary syndrome. Arch gynecol obstet. 2012;285(3):853-856.

28. Janssen OE, Mehlmauer N, Hahn S, Offner AH, Gartner R. High prevalence of autoimmune thyroiditis in patients with polycystic ovary syndrome. European J Endocrinol. 2004;150(3):363-369.

29. Boomsma CM, Eijkemans MJ, Hughes EG, Visser GH, Fauser BC, Macklon NS. A meta-analysis of pregnancy outcomes in women with polycystic ovary syndrome. Human reprod update. 2006;12(6):673-683.

30. Azziz R, Carmina E, Dewailly D, et al. Positions statement: criteria for defining polycystic ovary syndrome as a predominantly hyperandrogenic syndrome: an Androgen Excess Society guideline. J Clin Endocrinol Metab. 2006;91(11):4237-4245.

31. Toulis KA, Goulis DG, Mintziori G, et al. Meta-analysis of cardiovascular disease risk markers in women with polycystic ovary syndrome. Human reprod update. 2011;17(6):741-760.

32. Balen AH, Laven JS, Tan SL, Dewailly D. Ultrasound assessment of the polycystic ovary: international consensus definitions. Human reprod update. 2003;9(6):505-514.

33. Nieuwenhuis-Ruifrok AE, Kuchenbecker WK, Hoek A, Middleton P, Norman RJ. Insulin sensitizing drugs for weight loss in women of reproductive age who are overweight or obese: systematic review and meta-analysis. Human reprod update. 2009;15(1):57-68.

34. Palomba S, Falbo A, Zullo F, Orio F, Jr. Evidence-based and potential benefits of metformin in the polycystic ovary syndrome: a comprehensive review. Endocrine reviews. 2009;30(1):1-50.

35. Sherif K. Benefits and risks of oral contraceptives. Amer J Obst Gynecol. 1999;180(6 Pt 2):S343-348.

36. Lord JM, Flight IH, Norman RJ. Metformin in polycystic ovary syndrome: systematic review and meta-analysis. BMJ. 2003;327(7421):951-953.

37. Cheang KI, Huszar JM, Best AM, Sharma S, Essah PA, Nestler JE. Long-term effect of metformin on metabolic parameters in the polycystic ovary syndrome. Diabetes Vascular Dis. 2009;6(2):110-119.

38. Garber AJ, Duncan TG, Goodman AM, Mills DJ, Rohlf JL. Efficacy of

metformin in type II diabetes: results of a double-blind, placebo-controlled, dose-response trial. Amer J Med. 1997;103(6):491-497.

39. Colmers IN, Bowker SL, Majumdar SR, Johnson JA. Use of thiazolidinediones and the risk of bladder cancer among people with type 2 diabetes: a meta-analysis. CMAJ. 2012;184(12):E675-683.

Chapter 2

NUTRITIONAL STRATEGIES AND LIFESTYLE MODIFICATIONS FOR PCOS

By Lynn Monahan, DCN, MPH, RD, LDN
AND
Patricia G. Davidson, DCN, MS, RD, CDE

As the previous chapter described, PCOS is a chronic endocrine disorder with both reproductive and metabolic components. Research has advanced our understanding of PCOS' pathogenesis, specifically that insulin resistance is present in approximately 50% to 80% of women with the syndrome,[1] regardless of weight. This insulin resistance contributes to PCOS symptoms and increases the risk of developing metabolic syndrome,[2] cardiovascular disease (CVD), and T2DM[3] often found in women with PCOS. Insulin resistance causes the development of hyperinsulinemia,[4] which contributes to the metabolic abnormalities and elevated androgens observed in women with PCOS.[5] Thus, treatment aimed at lowering insulin levels and improving insulin sensitivity is key to managing the syndrome.

Evidence-based lifestyle interventions involving behavioral, dietary, and exercise management is the primary focus of treatment for women with PCOS.[6] Prescription medications, including insulin-sensitizing agents, and surgery may be used in combination or as adjunct treatment. Diet and exercise have been shown to successfully manage insulin resistance and weight loss, and improve reproduction and metabolic risk factors in the PCOS population.[4,7-1117]

Because lifestyle modification is an integral component of PCOS treatment, it's necessary for dietetics professionals to have adequate knowledge and training regarding PCOS physiology and medical nutrition therapy (MNT) strategies. This chapter presents the current evidence-based recommendations for lifestyle modifications for treating PCOS, including weight loss, specific dietary components, and exercise strategies. Applications and the dietitian's role in treating PCOS are also discussed.

WEIGHT LOSS AND PCOS

Although not all women with PCOS are overweight or obese, it's common for them to have a higher BMI; approximately 40% to 60% of PCOS patients have a high BMI.[12] In a systematic review of more than 15,000 women with PCOS, Lim et al found an increased prevalence of overweight, obesity, and abdominal obesity in this population compared with women without PCOS.[12] Androgen-associated weight gain increases abdominal visceral fat and has been observed in both overweight and lean women with PCOS.[13] Central obesity worsens both the reproductive and metabolic features of PCOS, primarily through increasing insulin resistance.[14] Because both obese and nonobese women with PCOS tend to have an intrinsic or PCOS-specific insulin resistance, weight loss and preventing weight gain is recommended as the first-line treatment.[15]

Studies have shown that overweight women with PCOS who lose as little as 5% to 10% of their initial body weight experience improved metabolic parameters (insulin resistance, hyperandrogenism, fasting glucose, and dyslipidemia) and reproductive features (menstrual function, ovulation, conception, and pregnancy rates).[6,16,17-18] This means that a woman with PCOS who weighs 220 lbs can expect to see improvements in her labs and symptoms plus experience more regular menstrual cycles if she loses 11 lbs.

Because weight loss improves nearly every aspect of PCOS, weight loss should be the primary goal for overweight women with PCOS. Individual variability with weight loss has been reported in PCOS. In a study by Pasquali et al, 65 women with PCOS who participated in an intervention program over six months achieved a greater than 5% sustained weight loss.[19] The researchers found that sustained weight loss resulted in a full recovery from PCOS features for 37% of the women (n = 24) and partial recovery for 48% (n = 31), while 15.4% (n = 10) still presented with PCOS despite comparable weight loss.

Interestingly, the larger the amount of abdominal fat at baseline, the less probability that lifestyle management and weight loss would improve the PCOS symptoms.

Although diet and lifestyle are the primary treatment approaches for addressing PCOS, specific dietary recommendations for women with PCOS have not been established. Controversy remains over the optimal diet composition because of limited literature, the lack of long-term randomized controlled trials (RCTs), and conflicting findings. Recommendations have been published for the general US population and include higher-fiber, low-fat, (approximately 30% of energy and 10% saturated fat with fewer than 300 mg of cholesterol), moderate-protein (approximately 15%), and higher-carbohydrate (approximately 55%) diets.[20] A systematic review of the effect of different dietary compositions on anthropometric, metabolic, reproductive, and psychological outcomes in PCOS found no differences between diet composition and weight loss.[27] Caloric (energy) restriction, rather than altered dietary composition, is most effective in achieving weight loss and improved clinical benefits. This review, however, included only five studies, only one of which was an RCT.

MACRONUTRIENT COMPOSITIONS

At this time, there is no clear optimal dietary strategy for treating PCOS. Subsequently, treatment strategies vary, focusing on macronutrient composition and type and hypocaloric diets as well as comprehensive lifestyle modification programs that include behavior modification, stress management, diet, and pharmacology. This requires dietitians to individualize diet guidelines based on each PCOS patient's needs and goals. If weight loss is recommended, nutrition counseling and education efforts should provide modifications for macronutrient distribution to best support caloric reductions for the individual patient while still meeting Dietary Reference Intakes (DRIs).

High-Protein Diets

A high-protein, low-carbohydrate diet traditionally has been thought to aid in weight loss and improve metabolic and reproductive dysfunction in PCOS.[21] Perhaps because of protein's satiating effect compared with carbohydrates or fat, or improving insulin sensitivity through the maintenance of lean body mass with weight loss, a high-protein, low-carbohydrate diet has been considered the premier dietary treatment for PCOS.[18]

A six-month RCT involving 57 women with PCOS showed the benefits of a high-protein diet (greater than 40% of calories from protein, 30% fat) on glucose metabolism, C-peptide production, and weight loss compared with the effects of a standard-protein diet (less than 15% protein, 30% fat).[22] The women were divided into two groups, neither of which was required to restrict calories. The high-protein diet resulted in greater loss of weight (7.7 kg vs. 3.3 kg) and body fat despite the lack of caloric reduction. Additionally, those following a high-protein diet saw greater reductions in waist circumference and decreases in glucose than those following the standard-protein diet. There were no differences in testosterone, SHBG, and blood lipids between the groups. The researchers suggested that the high-protein diet group lost more weight because of the satisfying effects of protein on appetite—that is, the women may have felt more satisfied and less hungry when eating a high-protein diet so that they consumed less food overall.

Chavarro et al found that the type of dietary protein influenced fertility. Consuming animal sources of protein was associated with a higher risk of ovulatory infertility, with a lower risk associated with the consumption of vegetable protein in place of carbohydrates or animal protein.[23]

Moran et al examined the effect of modifying dietary protein and carbohydrates on lipids and arterial compliance.[24] Twenty-eight women with PCOS who were overweight were randomized to a low-protein (16% protein, 57% carbohydrate) or high-protein (27% protein, 43% carbohydrate), hypocaloric diet for 12 weeks. The intervention period was followed by four weeks of an energy-balanced diet. Fasting insulin, triglycerides, fasting free fatty acids, and CRP all decreased as well as weight (7.7 ± 3.7 kg), with no significant difference between the dietary-specific groups. Weight loss benefitted arterial compliance (elasticity of blood vessels) through improvements in insulin resistance, inflammation, and blood pressure. Weight loss through caloric restriction improved fasting, postprandial lipids and arterial compliance, supporting the efficacy of weight loss in improving vascular indices in PCOS. However, this study did not find that modifying macronutrient composition influenced cardiovascular risk factors.

The amount and source of dietary protein and how it affects ovulatory function in PCOS remains unknown. While protein-rich foods do not cause the same immediate or degree of postprandial insulin release as seen with carbohydrates, it still elicits a response, though the effect remains unclear.[23,25,26] Protein intake can affect insulin and glucose differently depending on the type.[23] The postprandial insulin response to vegetable protein and eggs is lower than to red meat or other animal proteins.[27,28]

However, there are health risks associated with high-protein diets.[29] Typically, these diets include foods high in saturated fat and cholesterol (e.g, cheese, meat, eggs) and may be deficient in a number of vitamins, minerals, antioxidants, and fiber because of a limited intake of fruits, vegetables, and whole grains.[30,31] High-protein diets also could potentially negatively affect bone and kidney metabolism.[29] Feeding studies have shown that a high-protein, low-carbohydrate diet decreases vascular elasticity and potentially increases cardiovascular risk in the long-term.[32] Some people may experience hypoglycemia when avoiding carbohydrates, which can lead to binge eating and possibly contributing to the development of distorted eating or eating disorders (see Chapter 8). And some people simply cannot follow this type of diet for very long because of its rigidity.

Very Low-Calorie Diets and PCOS

Studies have shown very low-calorie diets to be effective for weight loss and improving reproductive and metabolic parameters in women with PCOS.[33-36] Sibutramine added to a hypocaloric diet for six months resulted in significant weight loss in women with PCOS who were overweight or obese, along with improvements in hyperandrogenemia and insulin sensitivity.[36]

Tolino et al examined the effect of long-term caloric restriction on both clinical and biochemical abnormalities in 114 women with PCOS who were obese.[34] The participants followed a strict low-calorie diet (500 kcal/day) for four weeks followed by 1,000 kcal/day for seven months. Fifty-four percent of the women lost more than 5% of body weight, while 11.8% remained at their pretreatment weight, demonstrating the difficulty women with PCOS have with weight loss.

Both groups experienced improvements in testosterone levels and in those who lost weight, there were significant improvements in blood insulin levels; 81.8% showed improvement in reproductive function.[34]

In a 12-week randomized pilot study, young women with PCOS (ages 12 to 22) followed a low-fat, low-calorie diet or a low-carbohydrate diet.[33] Both groups received nutrition counseling during the study, and there were no statistically significant differences between the groups.

Weight loss averaged 6.5%, and waist circumference decreased by an average of 5.7 ± 7.7 cm. Those who lost weight were 3.4 times more likely to have improved menstrual function.[33]

Another study compared the effects on weight loss of meal replacements followed by six months of dietary macronutrient restriction.[35] Forty-three women with PCOS who were overweight were provided meal replacements for two meals per day over eight weeks, then one-half of the subjects followed either a low-carbohydrate diet (fewer than 120 g/day) or a low-fat diet (fewer than 50 g/day) for 24 weeks. Meal replacements improved weight (5.6 ± 2.4 kg), waist circumference (6.1 ± 2.5 cm), body fat (4.1 ± 2.2 kg), insulin (2.8 ± 1.1 mU/L), total testosterone (0.3 ± 0.7 nmol/L), and free androgen index (3.1 ± 4.6). Both carbohydrate and fat restricted diets maintained weight loss and improved reproductive and metabolic variables following meal replacements.[35]

Meal replacements or very low calorie diets are effective strategies for short-term weight loss and improvement in PCOS features for some women. However, long-term adherence is extremely difficult. Those who experience dietary relapse will often regain weight,[37] which means the manifestations of PCOS and associated long-term morbidity and mortality risks are likely to return as well.[38]

The Glycemic Index Diet for Women with PCOS

Women with PCOS have a four times greater risk of developing T2DM than those without PCOS and have a 10-fold greater risk of developing CVD.[24] The glycemic index (GI) /glycemic load (GL) diet has been used in the PCOS population as an intervention to lower risk for these diseases, yet skepticism remains regarding the efficacy of low-GI/GL diets for decreasing the risk of T2DM or CVD and in weight loss or maintenance,[39] as many of the studies have ended with inconsistent findings.

In 2008, Hare-Bruun et al got mixed results when they reviewed the epidemiological literature on GI/GL and the effect on heart disease, T2DM, dyslipidemia, and obesity in a healthy adult population. There was a positive association between low GI and a decreased risk of T2DM. The women in the studies also experienced a reduced risk of heart disease, however, a reduction in heart-protective HDL cholesterol was also seen. The reviewers concluded there was not enough evidence to include GI/GL in dietary recommendations for the prevention of chronic disease.[40]

In contrast, also in 2008, Barclay et al completed a systematic review of 37 prospective cohort studies evaluating a low-GI/GL diet and the risk of chronic disease. The results provided evidence that a low-GI/GL diet may prevent the development of T2DM and CHD.[41]

The protective effect of a low-GI/GL diet on improving glycemic control was further supported by a meta-analysis by Thomas et al involving 11 RCTs that showed a low-GI diet can result in better glycemic control and decrease the number of hypoglycemic events compared with a high-GI diet.[42]

T2DM is characterized by insulin resistance, and studies have found that in healthy patients a low GI/GL diet preserved insulin sensitivity[43] or improved insulin sensitivity in those with prediabetes,[44] T2DM, or CHD, a low-GI/GL.[45] In a recent review of dietary GI and the risk of developing T2DM and CVD, seven of the 11 prospective epidemiologic studies reviewed demonstrated a positive association between a low-GI/GL diet and the risk of T2DM.[46]

A review by Esfahani et al examined 20 trials involving the GI/GL diet and its effect on weight loss.[47] The results revealed numerous inconsistencies, with four trials favoring a low-GI/GL diet, while 10 concluded that such a diet enhanced weight loss but not enough to be statistically significant. The remaining studies saw weight gain in both groups or another diet strategy result in greater weight loss.[47]

An interesting finding from this review indicated that a low-GI/GL diet may be more effective for weight loss and the reduction of body fat in people with elevated postprandial insulin levels or hyperinsulinemia,[48] which is common in the PCOS population. Ebbling et al also found that individuals with elevated baseline insulin levels lost more weight by following a low-GI intake (13 lbs vs. 3 lbs).[49]

Ludwig reported on 13 studies examining the effects of different GI diets with similar composition on serum lipids in individuals with hyperlipidemia and diabetes.[50] The majority of the studies demonstrated that a low-GI diet can decrease the ratio of triglycerides and LDL cholesterol and the ratio of total and HDL cholesterol.[50]

Whole grain consumption also has been linked to reducing the risk of CHD.[51] In the Framingham Offspring Cohort Heart Study, individuals consuming a diet high in GI/GL foods had higher rates of metabolic syndrome and insulin resistance.[51]

The Dietary Approaches to Stop Hypertension (DASH) study further exemplifies the benefits of a low-GI diet on CHD risk. Participants in the DASH study showed significant improvements in lipids and blood pressure despite a relatively high carbohydrate intake from fruits, vegetables, whole grain foods, and low-fat dairy products (57%).[52]

Studies examining the effects of low-GI/GL diets with metabolic and reproductive parameters in women with PCOS are limited. A group of British researchers completed a retrospective chart review of 59 PCOS patients who were overweight or lean and had been prescribed a low-GI/GL diet as part of a hypocaloric meal plan.[53] All participants were taking insulin-sensitizing medication after being diagnosed with insulin resistance.

At baseline, the majority of patients self-reported experiencing carbohydrate cravings, tiredness and lethargy, central weight gain, hunger, and symptoms of hypoglycemia. Follow-up data demonstrated a significant decrease in weight, BMI, and waist circumference in the overweight patients; fasting glucose decreased significantly but not fasting insulin levels. Fifty-two percent reported a decrease in carbohydrate cravings on the low-GI diet, and normal-weight women experienced markedly fewer hypoglycemic events (73% vs. 11%). Symptoms of hunger, tiredness, and lethargy were greatly reduced in both women who were overweight (54% vs. 29%) and lean (83% vs. 40%). The low-GI/GL diet contributed to the relief of symptoms commonly reported in women with PCOS.

Acne is common in women with PCOS, regardless of age. High-GL diets have been found to contribute to acne development in non-PCOS individuals by changing circulating hormone levels, binding proteins and receptors, leading to increased cellular growth and sebum production.[54] High-GL diets have also been shown to increase hyperinsulinemia, which stimulates insulin growth factor 1 (IGF-1), a powerful mediator of cellular and follicular growth, which in turn increases androgen production.[54] Interestingly, acne symptoms improved when individuals followed low-GL diets.[54]

In a nonrandomized control trial, Marsh et al compared the effects of a low-GI diet with a conventional diet (high fiber and moderate to high-GI breads and cereals) in 96 women with PCOS.[55] The participants consumed a low-GI diet or a macronutrient-matched healthy diet without caloric restriction for 12 months. Those who followed the low-GI diet had significantly increased menstrual regularity (95% vs. 63% on a conventional diet) and insulin sensitivity. Women who took metformin and followed the low-GI diet had the best improvement in insulin sensitivity. Those with high insulin levels at baseline experienced a twofold reduction in body fat despite modest weight loss compared with the conventional diet.[55]

Both the type and amount of carbohydrates in the diet are important for treating PCOS and ovulatory infertility.[56] Chavarro et al found that greater carbohydrate intake and GL were associated with anovulation in healthy women.[56]

Moderate amounts of carbohydrates, if in the low-GI form, can be beneficial for treating PCOS, as they can improve insulin sensitivity, glucose tolerance, hyperlipidemia, ovulation, and metabolic syndrome. Low-GI foods contain more fiber and take longer to chew, which tends to increase satiety, reduce hunger, and lower subsequent voluntary food intake. In contrast, high-GI foods have been known to increase androgen production[54] and stimulate appetite, leading to greater food intake.[25] Therefore, women with PCOS do not need to avoid carbohydrates, but the type and quantity they consume may need to be modified for optimal results.

Dietary Fat

Traditionally, low-fat diets were advised for weight loss, especially in improving metabolic syndrome in the general population.[31] However, according to Willet, short-term trials of low-fat diets resulted in minimal changes in body weight, and long-term trials (longer than one year) also resulted in little or no weight loss.[57] Research implies that a higher carbohydrate intake, particularly from refined carbohydrates, combined with a low-fat diet can actually make metabolic syndrome worse, as it can exaggerate postprandial glycemia and increase obesity.[48]

Focusing on low-fat, high-GI diets can be problematic, as they can increase triglyceride levels, decrease HDL concentrations, and negatively affect blood pressure.[31,58] Low-fat diet recommendations can inadvertently promote higher consumption of refined carbohydrates, especially because manufacturers tend to add sugar to reduced-fat products. Too little fat in the diet can also contribute to hunger, overeating, and weight gain, as fat contributes to satiety.[57]

Like carbohydrates, it appears that both the type of fat—saturated, polyunsaturated (PUFA), monounsaturated (MUFA), and trans—and amount are important. A high intake of saturated and trans fats has been found to cause dyslipidemia and hyperinsulinemia, increasing the risk of diabetes and metabolic syndrome.[31] Interestingly, when comparing diet composition for women with PCOS in the United States and Italy, caloric intake was similar, but women in the United States consumed more saturated fat and had a higher BMI.[59]

A 20-year follow-up study supported an inverse relationship between PUFA intake and CHD risk in women; trans fat intake was associated with an increased risk of CHD.[60] A large prospective study conducted on more than 80,000 women enrolled in the Nurses' Health Study found that substituting MUFAs and PUFAs for just 5% of saturated fat calories reduced the risk of CHD in women by 42%.[61]

In a study of reproductive function and insulin resistance in women who were hyperandrogenic and postmenopausal, Berrino et al modified participants' diets to be high in plant-based fats, low-GI foods, MUFAs, and omega-3 fatty acids.[62] Reduced insulin resistance, improved weight loss, and a significant decrease in waist-to-hip ratios were found, along with increases in SHBG and decreases in serum testosterone levels.[69]

It has been well documented that women with PCOS have high susceptibility for developing NAFLD.[63,64] Elevated triglycerides and insulin levels are contributing factors in the development of NAFLD. Because of the clinical association between PCOS and NAFLD, it is prudent to consider recommending women with PCOS supplement or substitute saturated fats with omega-3 fatty acids. A meta-analysis indicated the benefits of omega-3 fatty acids for treating fatty liver disease.[65]

Consumption of omega-3 fatty acids has been shown to decrease insulin resistance in women with PCOS.[65,66] Omega-3 fats benefit women with metabolic syndrome and T2DM as well as those with PCOS because of their ability to improve triglycerides, sex hormones,

LDL and HDL concentrations, and blood pressure.[67,68] The benefits of MUFAs and PUFAs for improving inflammation[68] and androgen levels[62,66,67] in PCOS also have been shown. In one study, 31 women with PCOS were randomized to receive for six weeks either walnuts (PUFAs) or almonds (MUFAs) containing 31 g of total fat per day. While no change in weight was observed, both almonds and walnuts reduced LDL cholesterol. Walnuts increased insulin response during an OGTT by 26% and decreased HbA1c from 5.7 ± 0.1 to $5.5 \pm 0.1\%$.[62] Walnuts increased SHBG, and almonds decreased free androgen levels. Researchers concluded that nut intake positively affects plasma lipids and androgens in women with PCOS.[62]

Dietary fat also may play an important role in fertility. A prospective cohort study of 18,555 premenopausal women showed that each 2% increase in energy from trans fats was associated with a 73% greater risk of ovulatory infertility.[69] Women with high scores on a "fertility diet," characterized by low trans fats with a greater intake of MUFAs, vegetable protein, fiber, low-GI carbohydrates, and high-fat dairy products, had a reduced risk of ovulatory infertility.[70]

While it is clear that omega-3 fats play an important role in the treatment of PCOS, therapeutic amounts have not been established. Women with PCOS who were not obese were given 1,500 mg of omega-3 fats daily for six months.[66] BMI plus insulin levels decreased significantly during treatment, but glucose levels did not change. Additionally, serum LH and testosterone levels decreased, and SHBG levels increased significantly. The researchers concluded that omega-3s also may be effective for improving hirsutism and insulin resistance in women with PCOS.[66]

Current National Cholesterol Education Panel Adult Treatment Plan III guidelines suggest daily total fat intake should range between 25% and 35%, while saturated fat intake should be limited to less than 7%. PUFAs should make up as much as 10% of total calories and MUFAs up to 20%.[71] To meet these requirements, government guidelines encourage Americans to consume fatty fish twice a week.[72] Each serving should be 3.5 oz cooked, or about ¾ cup of flaked fish. Fatty fish such as salmon, mackerel, herring, lake trout, sardines, and albacore tuna are high in omega-3 fatty acids.

Despite the possible benefits of a higher unsaturated fat diet for improving PCOS, not all experts agree on the exact macronutrient breakdown. A major concern of these diets is the possibility of weight gain because of the high caloric content of dietary fat. Even though the fat sources substituting for reduced carbohydrate intake would be MUFAs and PUFAs, the increase in fat content could increase the total calorie intake and may limit weight loss.

DAIRY AND PCOS

Research has shown that dairy consumption can impact fertility and acne development. A large prospective cohort of women without a history of infertility found that the type of dairy products they consumed influenced fertility. Low-fat dairy foods increased the risk of anovulatory infertility, whereas high-fat dairy foods decreased the risk.[73] According to the researchers, one explanation for this is that when the fat is taken out of milk, it alters the hormone balance of milk, including sex hormones, which in turn influence women's hormones.[74]

In a review of 27 studies, Burris et al found that frequent dairy intake (three or more servings of milk daily) contributed to acne, for example, because it can contribute to increased insulin levels, leading to increased cellular growth and acne. Milk has a high GL and contains growth-stimulating hormones, which stimulate IGF-1, resulting in hyperinsulinemia and increased androgens and subsequently higher sebum production.[54] Interestingly, acne was positively associated with the consumption of total milk or skim milk but not whole milk.

No RCTs have examined the relationship between milk or dairy consumption and acne. Most of the studies conducted have relied on self-reported dairy intake and focus on milk, not cheese or other dairy sources.[75,76] There are no formal guidelines regarding what type or how much dairy women with PCOS should consume or if it is necessary to avoid dairy. Because of the direct influence on andro-gens and insulin, it may be advisable for women with PCOS, regard-less of whether they have acne, to limit their dairy intake to two or fewer servings each day. If a woman is trying to conceive, moderate amounts of full-fat dairy sources may be advised.[74] Ultimately, dairy's role in PCOS requires further research.

Adult women need 1,000 mg of calcium daily. Other ways to get calcium, besides dairy products are, cow's milk alternatives (e.g., almond, hemp, rice, coconut), certain vegetables (e.g., kale, broccoli, bok choy), fish (5 oz of salmon contains more calcium than a glass of milk), and seeds (e.g., chia, sesame, flax).

GLUTEN AND PCOS

Perform an Internet search on nutrition for PCOS and you will be sure to come across websites promoting a gluten-free diet. For the 1% of people diagnosed with celiac disease, and the small percentage who have nonceliac gluten sensitivity, strict adherence to a gluten-free diet is crucial. Avoiding gluten can help these individuals feel better and experience less symptoms, such as bloating, abdominal pain, and fatigue.

PCOS is a state of inflammation correlated with insulin resistance. Women with PCOS have higher CRP values, independent of BMI.[77] It has been suggested that the daily consumption of wheat products and other related cereal grains may contribute to chronic inflammation and autoimmune diseases.[78] Reducing gluten consumption or avoiding it therefore could lessen inflammation in PCOS. A double-blind RCT examined the effects of dietary gluten on inflammation in individuals with irritable bowel syndrome. Participants who received gluten reported significantly more symptoms compared with the placebo group.[79] No significant changes in CRP levels were observed.

Despite the Internet showing the popularity of gluten-free diets for PCOS, there are no evidence-based studies confirming their efficacy for treating the syndrome. It is common for individuals who adopt a gluten-free diet to have a lower carbohydrate or caloric intake, which can result in weight loss and improve symptoms of PCOS. For example, gluten-free high-fiber whole grains such as quinoa and brown rice are low-GI foods.

However, a gluten-free diet has some disadvantages. If not followed correctly, it can result in iron, folate, niacin, zinc, and fiber deficiencies. Many gluten-free foods have added sugars to maintain flavor. Gluten-free diets can result in weight gain, as products sometimes contain more calories and sugar than their gluten-containing counterparts. For example, a single serving of regular pretzels provides 108 kcal, but a serving of gluten-free pretzels has 140 kcal.

Dietitians should carefully screen women with PCOS for celiac disease or nonceliac gluten sensitivity. If a sensitivity is suspected, after having been medically tested for celiac disease, dietitians may instruct women to follow a gluten-free elimination diet, after which small amounts of gluten-containing foods can be gradually reintroduced. If a patient does have gluten sensitivity, she will feel significantly better following a gluten-free diet. Research examining the relationship between gluten and PCOS is needed.

BARRIERS TO CHANGE

Despite the benefits of weight loss, losing weight and maintaining weight loss is difficult in the general population and for women with PCOS.[80] Women with PCOS drop out of weight-loss studies at a higher rate (26% to 38%) compared with women without PCOS (8% to 9%).[81-83] Weight gain, especially in the abdominal region,[91,92] stimulates fat deposition and suppresses fat breakdown (lipolysis), spurring insulin resistance and hyperinsulinemia. As discussed next, women with PCOS commonly report increased cravings for high-fat and high-GI foods, and may have impaired appetite-regulating hormones. These factors combined can be barriers to lifestyle changes.

Food Cravings
Elevated insulin levels act as an appetite stimulant, increasing food cravings, especially for high-GI foods[58,84] and possibly carbohydrates. Lim et al studied the relationship of food cravings to hyperandrogenemia in 198 young, overweight non-PCOS women enrolled in a weight-loss program.[93] The participants craved chocolate more than any other food, along with carbohydrate-rich sweets and fast food. Those with menstrual disturbances had high overall food cravings, and those with hyperandrogenemia reported high-fat food cravings.

Other researchers found that the diet composition of PCOS women vs. non-PCOS women of the same BMI, race, and age group was essentially the same in regard to total energy and macronutrient intake, but women with PCOS consumed a higher amount of total fat and high-GI foods.[85] The women with PCOS also had hyperinsulinemia. The researchers concluded that women with PCOS do not necessarily eat more food but may eat a diet composed of higher amounts of simple carbohydrates and fat, possibly because of elevated insulin levels. Thus, higher protein intake may reduce cravings in women with PCOS because of its satiating effects.

Impaired Appetite Regulation

Another possible mechanism that could make weight loss and weight maintenance difficult for women with PCOS is hormonal influences that regulate appetite and satiety. Ghrelin is a hormone secreted from cells in the GI tract, primarily in the stomach, that increases preprandially to stimulate appetite and food intake and decreases postprandially, stimulating satiety. Ghrelin also plays a role in the regulation of energy balance, insulin levels, and glucose metabolism.[86]

Studies have provided evidence that pre- and postprandial ghrelin may be impaired in the PCOS population.[87,88] This is supported by a study by Bik et al that examined fasting ghrelin levels in 20 nonobese women with PCOS; 45 lean, healthy women; and 37 obese, non-PCOS women.[98] Fasting ghrelin levels were highest in the nonobese PCOS women and lowest in the women who were obese.

Significantly higher fasting ghrelin levels were found at baseline in an eight-week weight-loss study by Moran et al, who examined appetite hormones, including ghrelin, in 14 women with PCOS and 14 without PCOS.[89] The participants followed a hypocaloric diet with meal replacements for two meals. There were no differences in weight loss between the groups (4.2 kg vs. 4.3 kg), and both groups had lowered postprandial plasma ghrelin. However, the expected decrease of ghrelin levels was less in the PCOS group than the control group.

In addition to ghrelin, cholecystokinin (CCK) levels have been found to be dysfunctional in women with PCOS.[89,90] CCK, a hormone secreted by the small intestine, is released postprandially in response to protein and fat in the duodenum, inhibiting gastric emptying and signaling satiety. When matched with controls, women with PCOS who were overweight were found to have reduced postprandial CCK response.[89,90] While it is not known why women with PCOS have impaired CCK secretion following meals, it has been suggested that they may have delayed gastric emptying.[90]

Leptin, which is involved in energy balance and reproduction, may be implicated in the pathogenesis of PCOS.[91] There is a positive correlation between leptin and BMI as well as leptin and testosterone in women with PCOS.[92] Kedikova et al showed adolescent girls with PCOS who had increased adipose tissue had significantly higher serum leptin levels compared with healthy controls. Additionally, leptin was significantly higher in PCOS cases than in controls (39.9 ± 4.6 vs. 26.4 ± 3.4) among a sample of Bahraini women.[91] Decreased leptin function may stimulate hunger in women with PCOS, resulting in increased food intake and difficulty managing weight. In addition, having impaired levels of CCK and ghrelin could also explain why women with PCOS cannot lose weight: appetite signals are compromised, making them hungrier and leading to higher calorie consumption.

EXERCISE AND PCOS

Physical activity has long been accepted as a key strategy in weight management and the overall maintenance of physical and emotional health. Regular exercise is predictive of weight loss and long-term weight maintenance.[93] It is well established that exercise improves a number of health-related outcomes in the general population, such as dyslipidemia, hypertension, and insulin resistance, with an overall decrease in the risk of developing CVD and T2DM.[94] Exercise leads to psychological improvements in mood, self-esteem, and overall feelings of well-being.[95]

The 2008 Physical Activity Guidelines for Americans advises adults to engage in at least 150 minutes of moderate physical activity per week for substantial health benefits. For more extensive health benefits, aerobic activities should increase to 300 minutes per week. In addition, muscle strengthening should be done two or more times each week.[96] Intermittent exercise (10 to 15-minute increments) throughout the day can be just as effective as continuous exercise and may facilitate greater compliance for women with PCOS who perceive continuous physical activity as a barrier to exercising regularly.[96]

Although exercise is included in the lifestyle management recommendation for PCOS,[97] there are few exercise-specific RCTs involving the PCOS population, especially among lean women.[11] Studies that have examined the effects of exercise either alone or combination with caloric restriction demonstrated improved fitness, cardiovascular, hormonal, reproductive, and psychological outcomes.[10,11,98,99] Tomson et al demonstrated that while exercise did not lead to improvements in cardiometabolic risk factors, hormonal status, and reproductive function when added to a low-calorie diet for overweight women with PCOS, exercise did provide beneficial changes in body composition, including a 45% greater reduction in fat mass and a 60%

better preservation of fat-free mass (FFM).[23] Preservation of FFM, and thus resting metabolic rate (RMR), has potentially important implications for long-term weight-loss maintenance.[17]

Regular exercise may improve insulin sensitivity in PCOS, independent of weight loss.[98] Nineteen sedentary women with PCOS and insulin resistance who participated in a three-month exercise program showed a 25% improvement in insulin sensitivity and lipoprotein levels without significant weight loss.[100] The monitored program involved moderate-intensity exercise equivalent to walking briskly for one hour four days per week.

These results were supported by Harrison et al, who performed a systematic review to identify studies that examined the effect of exercise, independent of diet or other interventions, on the clinical outcomes of PCOS.[7] All eight of the studies reviewed (five RCTs and three cohorts) included moderate exercise levels and a longer duration (12 to 24 weeks). However, the type of exercise used varied considerably. Results demonstrated reduced insulin resistance (from 9% to 30%), overall weight loss of 4.5% to 10%, and improved ovulation.

Regular aerobic exercise has been shown to positively impact fertility in women with PCOS.[11,70] Women with PCOS who were obese and experiencing anovulatory infertility underwent a structured exercise training program that involved riding a stationary bicycle for 30 minutes three days per week or following a hypocaloric diet (800 kcal deficit consisting of 35% protein, 45% carbohydrate, and 20% fat) for 24 weeks.[99] While both groups showed improvements in menstrual cycles and fertility, the frequency of menses and the ovulation rates were significantly higher in the structured exercise training group than in the diet group. Body weight, BMI, waist circumference, insulin resistance indexes, and serum androgen levels changed significantly among both groups; however, the structured exercise training group showed better insulin resistance indexes.[99]

An RCT showed that a six-week intervention using the same structured exercise training program and hypocaloric diet modifications was effective for increasing the likelihood of ovulation with clomiphene citrate (Clomid) in overweight and obese women with PCOS who were Clomid resistant.[10] A small pilot study showed that exercise (one hour three days per week) without caloric restriction improved ovarian hormones in anovulatory overweight women with PCOS. [98]

Decreases in BMI, total fat mass, and improved insulin sensitivity were also shown.[98]

Researchers suggest that structured exercise training could improve insulin sensitivity and fertility not only for improving body weight reduction but also through cellular muscle metabolism enhancement.[99] Skeletal muscle is the main site of glucose deposition implicated in insulin resistance. Exercise influences the activity of proteins involved in insulin signal transduction in skeletal muscle.[99]

While aerobic exercise has been shown to benefit energy expenditure, strength training can be equally beneficial, as it can increase RMR and preserve or increase lean body mass. Strength training may be seen as a preferred choice for physical activity, especially among those with negative views toward traditional exercise. Additionally, moderate strength training, when combined with aerobic exercise (at 60–75% of heart rate), resulted in a greater improvement of insulin sensitivity than with aerobic exercise alone in postmenopausal women with type 2 diabetes.[101] Improvements in insulin indexes may result from reduced abdominal and visceral fat and the improvement of lean body mass.[101]

It has been demonstrated that women with PCOS, because they have higher androgen concentrations, have greater muscle strength than women without the syndrome.[102] Since muscle does weigh more than fat, it may be advisable for dietitians to use body composition measurements, including waist circumference, instead of relying on the scale to measure weight loss. For example, one client reportedly lost two dress sizes after three months of regular exercise that included strength training yet saw no difference in her weight.

Evidence clearly demonstrates the importance of physical activity for women with PCOS, regardless of weight status. Women with PCOS need to be educated on the benefits of regular physical activity for health and weight management. The use of motivational interviewing can be an effective behavior modification technique used to overcome perceived barriers to exercise, set realistic goals, and reinforce exercise patterns. Dietitians should encourage clients to engage in aerobic and strength training exercises that are acceptable and physically comfortable for them. Ideally, activities should be viewed as fun and enjoyable to encourage long-term compliance such as tennis, kayaking, biking, or walking. Increasing daily activities, such as climbing stairs instead of taking an elevator, parking the car further away from a destination, and walking down the hall to speak with a coworker instead of e-mailing him or her, for example, should also be encouraged. Some people find wearing a pedometer with a daily goal of 10,000 steps (approximately 4 to 5 miles), motivating to increase activity.

THE DIETITIAN'S ROLE IN RECOGNIZING AND TREATING PCOS

Early detection and treatment of PCOS is crucial because it can prevent excess weight gain, reduce the risk of chronic disease later in life, and lessen the emotional and financial burden of infertility. In a study on the effects of exercise and nutritional counseling on women with PCOS, Bruner et al found that nutritional counseling, with or without exercise, decreased insulin levels and improved both metabolic and reproductive abnormalities associated with PCOS.[103]

In working with their female patients, dietitians have the opportunity to identify those with a higher risk of obesity-related metabolic and reproductive disturbances and provide effective MNT strategies.

The nutrition assessment is the optimal time to screen all female clients for PCOS. Asking questions such as "Tell me what your periods are like. Are they heavy? Irregular?" or "Do you struggle with excessive body hair?" may reveal signs of PCOS that could require further testing. (Additional screening questions can be found in the Appendix.)

Diet modifications should be individualized according to clients' symptoms, health concerns, knowledge, past history with dieting, eating preferences, and readiness to change. According to Moran et al, because of "inconsistent differences in dietary compositions, it may be better to focus on the importance of increasing engagement, adherence, and sustainability with lifestyle change rather than the diet itself."[29]

In addition to exploring clients' eating habits and attitudes toward food and weight, dietitians should review laboratory tests with them (see Chapter 1 for information on these and other labs used to diagnose and treat PCOS). Lab results can be a great motivational tool for clients to monitor metabolic improvements as they make changes to their eating patterns and activity levels.

Not only do clients need dietitians to educate them on healthful, balanced diets, but they also need to be educated on the pathophysiology of PCOS. Clients need to understand how the hormonal imbalance of PCOS affects their symptoms as well as the increased risk of heart disease and diabetes. Education should include insulin's role in the body, what insulin resistance is, how insulin affects weight, the benefits of exercise, and how both the type and quantity of food affects insulin levels. The benefits and risks of dietary supplements to improve PCOS may also be discussed (see Chapter 3). The use of food models, food journaling and label reading, anthropometric measurements, and the scale are all helpful tools dietitians can use to provide effective nutrition education and monitoring to women with PCOS and are discussed in the Appendix.

Dietitians should take an empathetic approach in counseling their PCOS clients. Many women are embarrassed and frustrated about their symptoms. It could be helpful to let clients know they are not alone in their diagnosis and that the symptoms they experience, including their struggles with weight, are common among the PCOS population. It is also common for these women to feel hopeless, so they need to know that changes in diet and lifestyle can make a difference in reproductive and metabolic aspects, even if not accompanied by weight loss.

If necessary, dietitians can refer clients to therapists with experience in PCOS for mental health treatment and, if available, PCOS support groups. Ultimately, clients' readiness, knowledge, and understanding of their diagnosis should dictate the direction of nutrition sessions, including nutrition education and goal setting.

In summary, the primary treatment for PCOS is a combination of lifestyle modifications through diet and exercise. MNT plays an integral role in preventing and treating the clinical manifestations associated with PCOS as well as improving reproductive function. The optimal diet for PCOS is one that reduces negative metabolic consequences, improves ovulation, and decreases the risk of chronic disease. Weight loss has been shown to improve metabolic, reproductive, and psychological aspects of PCOS irrespective of diet composition. Dietitians should take an empathetic and supportive approach when counseling women with PCOS. Education of the syndrome's pathophysiology along with knowledge of how food affects insulin and glucose levels can be helpful to facilitate behavior changes.

CHAPTER SUMMARY

- Diet and lifestyle are considered the first-line approach for treating PCOS.
- The optimal diet composition for PCOS is unknown.
- Nutritional factors influence fertility.
- Weight loss improves both reproductive and metabolic parameters of PCOS. Weight loss or prevention of excess weight gain should be the main treatment consideration for women with PCOS.
- Very low-carbohydrate diets have not been proven to be superior to other diets in improving PCOS.
- Low-GI/GL diets offer numerous benefits for women with PCOS, including improved insulin and menstrual regularity, and weight loss.
- Dietitians need to educate women with PCOS on foods' effect on glucose and insulin levels.
- Omega-3-rich foods should be substituted for saturated and trans fats while keeping the total fat content to under 35% of total calories.
- Dairy intake should be limited to two servings or fewer per day to reduce acne, androgens, and insulin.
- Women with PCOS have been shown to have impaired appetite-regulating hormones.
- Both aerobic and resistance training have been shown to improve insulin sensitivity, body composition, and reproduction in women with PCOS.

REFERENCES

1. Legro RS, Castracane VD, Kauffman RP. Detecting insulin resistance in polycystic ovary syndrome: purposes and pitfalls. Obstet Gynecol Surv. 2004;59(2):141-154.

2. Apridonidze T, Essah PA, Iuorno MJ, Nestler JE. Prevalence and characteristics of the metabolic syndrome in women with polycystic ovary syndrome. J Clin Endocrinol Metab. 2005;90(4):1929-1935.

3. Goodarzi MO, Dumesic DA, Chazenbalk G, Azziz R. Polycystic ovary syndrome: etiology, pathogenesis and diagnosis. Nat Rev Endocrinol. 2011;7(4):219-231.

4. Giallauria F, Palomba S, Vigorito C, et al. Androgens in polycystic ovary syndrome: the role of exercise and diet. Semin Reprod Med. 2009;27(4):306-315.

5. Codner E, Escobar-Morreale HF. Clinical review: Hyperandrogenism and polycystic ovary syndrome in women with type 1 diabetes mellitus. J Clin Endocrinol Metab. 2007;92(4):1209-1216.

6. Moran LJ, Pasquali R, Teede HJ, Hoeger KM, Norman RJ. Treatment of obesity in polycystic ovary syndrome: a position statement of the Androgen Excess and Polycystic Ovary Syndrome Society. Fertil Steril. 2009;92(6):1966-1982.

7. Harrison CL, Lombard CB, Moran LJ, Teede HJ. Exercise therapy in polycystic ovary syndrome: a systematic review. Hum Reprod Update. 2011;17(2):171-183.

8. Harrison CL, Stepto NK, Hutchison SK, Teede HJ. The impact of intensified exercise training on insulin resistance and fitness in overweight and obese women with and without polycystic ovary syndrome. Clin Endocrinol. 2012;76(3):351-357.

9. Hutchison SK, Stepto NK, Harrison CL, Moran LJ, Strauss BJ, Teede HJ. Effects of exercise on insulin resistance and body composition in overweight and obese women with and without polycystic ovary syndrome. J Clin Endocrinol Metab. 2011;96(1):E48-56.

10. Palomba S, Falbo A, Giallauria F, et al. Six weeks of structured exercise training and hypocaloric diet increases the probability of ovulation after clomiphene citrate in overweight and obese patients with polycystic ovary syndrome: a randomized controlled trial. Hum Reprod. 2010;25(11):2783-2791.

11. Thomson RL, Buckley JD, Brinkworth GD. Exercise for the treatment and management of overweight women with polycystic ovary syndrome: a review of the literature. Obes. Rev. 2011;12(5):e202-210.

12. Lim SS, Davies MJ, Norman RJ, Moran LJ. Overweight, obesity and central obesity in women with polycystic ovary syndrome: a systematic review and meta-analysis. Hum Reprod Update. 2012.
13. Yildirim B, Sabir N, Kaleli B. Relation of intra-abdominal fat distribution to metabolic disorders in nonobese patients with polycystic ovary syndrome. Fertil Steril. 2003;79(6):1358-1364.
14. Liepa GU, Sengupta A, Karsies D. Polycystic ovary syndrome (PCOS) and other androgen excess-related conditions: can changes in dietary intake make a difference? Nut Clin Pract. 2008;23(1):63-71.
15. Teede HJ, Meyer C, Hutchison SK, Zoungas S, McGrath BP, Moran LJ. Endothelial function and insulin resistance in polycystic ovary syndrome: the effects of medical therapy. Fertil Steril. 2010;93(1):184-191.
16. Clark AM, Ledger W, Galletly C, et al. Weight loss results in significant improvement in pregnancy and ovulation rates in anovulatory obese women. Hum Reprod. 1995;10(10):2705-2712.
17. Thomson RL, Buckley JD, Noakes M, Clifton PM, Norman RJ, Brinkworth GD. The effect of a hypocaloric diet with and without exercise training on body composition, cardiometabolic risk profile, and reproductive function in overweight and obese women with polycystic ovary syndrome. J. Clin Endocrinol Metab. 2008;93(9):3373-3380.
18. Moran LJ, Noakes M, Clifton PM, Tomlinson L, Galletly C, Norman RJ. Dietary composition in restoring reproductive and metabolic physiology in overweight women with polycystic ovary syndrome. J Clin Endocrinol Metab. 2003;88(2):812-819.
19. Pasquali R, Gambineri A, Cavazza C, et al. Heterogeneity in the responsiveness to long-term lifestyle intervention and predictability in obese women with polycystic ovary syndrome. Eur J Endocrinol. 2011;164(1):53-60.
20. Clinical Guidelines on the Identification, Evaluation, and Treatment of Overweight and Obesity in Adults--The Evidence Report. National Institutes of Health. Obes Res. 1998;6 Suppl 2:51S-209S.
21. Moran LJ, Brinkworth G, Noakes M, Norman RJ. Effects of lifestyle modification in polycystic ovarian syndrome. Reprod Biomed Online. 2006;12(5):569-578.
22. Sorensen LB, Soe M, Halkier KH, Stigsby B, Astrup A. Effects of increased dietary protein-to-carbohydrate ratios in women with polycystic ovary syndrome. Am J Clin Nutr. 2012;95(1):39-48.
23. Chavarro JE, Rich-Edwards JW, Rosner BA, Willett WC. Protein intake and ovulatory infertility. Am J Obstet Gynecol. 2008;198(2):210 e211-217.

24. Moran LJ, Noakes M, Clifton PM, Norman RJ. The effect of modifying dietary protein and carbohydrate in weight loss on arterial compliance and postprandial lipidemia in overweight women with polycystic ovary syndrome. Fertil Steril. 2010;94(6):2451-2454.

25. Marsh K, Brand-Miller J. The optimal diet for women with polycystic ovary syndrome? Br J Nutr. 2005;94(2):154-165.

26. Moran LJ, Noakes M, Clifton PM, et al. Ghrelin and measures of satiety are altered in polycystic ovary syndrome but not differentially affected by diet composition. J Clin Endocrinol Metab. 2004;89(7):3337-3344.

27. Gannon MC, Nuttall FQ, Neil BJ, Westphal SA. The insulin and glucose responses to meals of glucose plus various proteins in type II diabetic subjects. Metabolism. 1988;37(11):1081-1088.

28. Hubbard R, Kosch CL, Sanchez A, Sabate J, Berk L, Shavlik G. Effect of dietary protein on serum insulin and glucagon levels in hyper- and normocholesterolemic men. Atherosclerosis. 1989;76(1):55-61.

29. Moran LJ, Ko H, Misso M, et al. Dietary composition in the treatment of polycystic ovary syndrome: a systematic review to inform evidence-based guidelines. J Acad Nutr Diet. 2013;113(4):520-545.

30. Kasim-Karakas SE, Cunningham WM, Tsodikov A. Relation of nutrients and hormones in polycystic ovary syndrome. Am J Clin Nutr. 2007;85(3):688-694.

31. Feldeisen SE, Tucker KL. Nutritional strategies in the prevention and treatment of metabolic syndrome. Appl Physiol Nutr Metab. 2007;32(1):46-60.

32. Bradley U, Spence M, Courtney CH, et al. Low-fat versus low-carbohydrate weight reduction diets: effects on weight loss, insulin resistance, and cardiovascular risk: a randomized control trial. Diabetes. 2009;58(12):2741-2748.

33. Ornstein RM, Copperman NM, Jacobson MS. Effect of weight loss on menstrual function in adolescents with polycystic ovary syndrome. J Pediatr Adolesc Gynecol. 2011;24(3):161-165.

34. Tolino A, Gambardella V, Caccavale C, et al. Evaluation of ovarian functionality after a dietary treatment in obese women with polycystic ovary syndrome. Eur J Obstet Gynecol Reprod Biol. 2005;119(1):87-93.

35. Moran LJ, Noakes M, Clifton PM, Wittert GA, Williams G, Norman RJ. Short-term meal replacements followed by dietary macronutrient restriction enhance weight loss in polycystic ovary syndrome. Am J Clin Nutr. 2006;84(1):77-87.

36. Florakis D, Diamanti-Kandarakis E, Katsikis I, et al. Effect of hypocaloric diet plus sibutramine treatment on hormonal and metabolic features in overweight and obese women with polycystic ovary syndrome: a randomized, 24-week study.

Int J Obes. 2008;32(4):692-699.

37. Moran LJ, Lombard CB, Lim S, Noakes M, Teede HJ. Polycystic ovary syndrome and weight management. Womens Health. 2010;6(2):271-283.

38. Norman RJ, Davies MJ, Lord J, Moran LJ. The role of lifestyle modification in polycystic ovary syndrome. Trends Endocrinol Metab. 2002;13(6):251-257.

39. van Bakel MM, Slimani N, Feskens EJ, et al. Methodological challenges in the application of the glycemic index in epidemiological studies using data from the European Prospective Investigation into Cancer and Nutrition. J Nutr. 2009;139(3):568-575.

40. Hare-Bruun H, Nielsen BM, Grau K, Oxlund AL, Heitmann BL. Should glycemic index and glycemic load be considered in dietary recommendations? Nutr Rev. 2008;66(10):569-590.

41. Barclay AW, Petocz P, McMillan-Price J, et al. Glycemic index, glycemic load, and chronic disease risk--a meta-analysis of observational studies. Am J Clin Nutr. 2008;87(3):627-637.

42. Thomas D, Elliott EJ. Low glycaemic index, or low glycaemic load, diets for diabetes mellitus. Cochrane Database Syst Rev. 2009(1):CD006296.

43. Pereira MA, Jacobs DR, Jr., Pins JJ, et al. Effect of whole grains on insulin sensitivity in overweight hyperinsulinemic adults. Am J Clin Nutr. 2002;75(5):848-855.

44. Wolever TM, Mehling C, Chiasson JL, et al. Low glycaemic index diet and disposition index in type 2 diabetes (the Canadian trial of carbohydrates in diabetes): a randomised controlled trial. Diabetologia. 2008;51(9):1607-1615.

45. Laaksonen DE, Toppinen LK, Juntunen KS, et al. Dietary carbohydrate modification enhances insulin secretion in persons with the metabolic syndrome. Am J Clin Nutr. 2005;82(6):1218-1227.

46. Chiu CJ, Liu S, Willett WC, et al. Informing food choices and health outcomes by use of the dietary glycemic index. Nutr Rev. 2011;69(4):231-242.

47. Esfahani A, Wong JM, Mirrahimi A, Villa CR, Kendall CW. The application of the glycemic index and glycemic load in weight loss: A review of the clinical evidence. IUBMB Life. 2011;63(1):7-13.

48. McMillan-Price J, Petocz P, Atkinson F, et al. Comparison of 4 diets of varying glycemic load on weight loss and cardiovascular risk reduction in overweight and obese young adults: a randomized controlled trial. Arch Intern Med. 2006;166(14):1466-1475.

49. Ebbeling CB, Leidig MM, Feldman HA, Lovesky MM, Ludwig DS. Effects of a low-glycemic load vs low-fat diet in obese young adults: a randomized trial. JAMA. 2007;297(19):2092-2102.

50. Ludwig DS. The glycemic index: physiological mechanisms relating to

obesity, diabetes, and cardiovascular disease. JAMA. 2002;287(18):2414-2423.

51. McKeown NM, Meigs JB, Liu S, Saltzman E, Wilson PW, Jacques PF. Carbohydrate nutrition, insulin resistance, and the prevalence of the metabolic syndrome in the Framingham Offspring Cohort. Diabetes Care. 2004;27(2):538-546.

52. Chen ST, Maruthur NM, Appel LJ. The effect of dietary patterns on estimated coronary heart disease risk: results from the Dietary Approaches to Stop Hypertension (DASH) trial. Circ. Cardiovasc Qual Outcomes. 2010;3(5):484-489.

53. Herriot AM, Whitcroft S, Jeanes Y. An retrospective audit of patients with polycystic ovary syndrome: the effects of a reduced glycaemic load diet. J Hum Nutr Diet. 2008;21(4):337-345.

54. Burris J, Rietkerk W, Woolf K. Acne: the role of medical nutrition therapy. J Acad Nutr Diet. 2013;113(3):416-430.

55. Marsh KA, Steinbeck KS, Atkinson FS, Petocz P, Brand-Miller JC. Effect of a low glycemic index compared with a conventional healthy diet on polycystic ovary syndrome. Am J Clin Nutr. 2010;92(1):83-92.

56. Chavarro JE, Rich-Edwards JW, Rosner BA, Willett WC. A prospective study of dietary carbohydrate quantity and quality in relation to risk of ovulatory infertility. Eur J Clin Nutr. 2009;63(1):78-86.

57. Willett WC. Dietary fat plays a major role in obesity: no. Obes Rev. 2002;3(2):59-68.

58. Moran L, Norman RJ. Understanding and managing disturbances in insulin metabolism and body weight in women with polycystic ovary syndrome. Best Pract Res Clin Obstet Gynaecol. 2004;18(5):719-736.

59. Carmina E, Legro RS, Stamets K, Lowell J, Lobo RA. Difference in body weight between American and Italian women with polycystic ovary syndrome: influence of the diet. Hum Reprod. 2003;18(11):2289-2293.

60. Oh K, Hu FB, Manson JE, Stampfer MJ, Willett WC. Dietary fat intake and risk of coronary heart disease in women: 20 years of follow-up of the nurses' health study. Am J Epidemiol. 2005;161(7):672-679.

61. Hu FB, Bronner L, Willett WC, et al. Fish and omega-3 fatty acid intake and risk of coronary heart disease in women. JAMA. 2002;287(14):1815-1821.

62. Berrino F, Bellati C, Secreto G, et al. Reducing bioavailable sex hormones through a comprehensive change in diet: the diet and androgens (DIANA) randomized trial. Cancer Epidemiol Biomarkers Prev. 2001;10(1):25-33.

63. Baranova A, Tran TP, Birerdinc A, Younossi ZM. Systematic review: association of polycystic ovary syndrome with metabolic syndrome and non-alcoholic fatty

liver disease. Aliment Pharmacol Ther. 2011;33(7):801-814.

64. Gambarin-Gelwan M, Kinkhabwala SV, Schiano TD, Bodian C, Yeh HC, Futterweit W. Prevalence of nonalcoholic fatty liver disease in women with polycystic ovary syndrome. Clin Gastroenterol Hepatol. 2007;5(4):496-501.

65. Parker HM, Johnson NA, Burdon CA, Cohn JS, O'Connor HT, George J. Omega-3 supplementation and non-alcoholic fatty liver disease: a systematic review and meta-analysis. J Hepatol. 2012;56(4):944-951.

66. Oner G, Muderris, II. Efficacy of omega-3 in the treatment of polycystic ovary syndrome. J. Obstet Gynaecol. 2013;33(3):289-291.

67. Phelan N, O'Connor A, Kyaw Tun T, et al. Hormonal and metabolic effects of polyunsaturated fatty acids in young women with polycystic ovary syndrome: results from a cross-sectional analysis and a randomized, placebo-controlled, crossover trial. Am J Clin Nutr. 2011;93(3):652-662.

68. Kalgaonkar S, Almario RU, Gurusinghe D, et al. Differential effects of walnuts vs almonds on improving metabolic and endocrine parameters in PCOS. Eur J Clin Nutr. 2011;65(3):386-393.

69. Chavarro JE, Rich-Edwards JW, Rosner BA, Willett WC. Dietary fatty acid intakes and the risk of ovulatory infertility. Am J Clin Nutr. 2007;85(1):231-237.

70. Chavarro JE, Rich-Edwards JW, Rosner BA, Willett WC. Diet and lifestyle in the prevention of ovulatory disorder infertility. Obstet Gynecol. 2007;110(5):1050-1058.

71. Third Report of the National Cholesterol Education Program (NCEP) Expert Panel on Detection, Evaluation, and Treatment of High Blood Cholesterol in Adults (Adult Treatment Panel III) final report. Circulation. 2002;106(25):3143-3421.

72. Kris-Etherton PM, Harris WS, Appel LJ. Fish consumption, fish oil, omega-3 fatty acids, and cardiovascular disease. Arterioscler Thromb Vasc Biol. 2003;23(2):e20-30.

73. Chavarro JE, Rich-Edwards JW, Rosner B, Willett WC. A prospective study of dairy foods intake and anovulatory infertility. Hum Reprod. 2007;22(5):1340-1347.

74. Chavarro J, Willet, W. The Fertility Diet. New York, NY: McGraw Hill; 2007.

75. Danby FW. Nutrition and acne. Clin Dermatol. 2010;28(6):598-604.

76. Adebamowo CA, Spiegelman D, Danby FW, Frazier AL, Willett WC, Holmes MD. High school dietary dairy intake and teenage acne. J Am Acad Dermatol. 2005;52(2):207-214.

77. El-Mesallamy HO, Abd El-Razek RS, El-Refaie TA. Circulating high-sensitivity C-reactive protein and soluble CD40 ligand are inter-related in a

cohort of women with polycystic ovary syndrome. Eur J Obstet Gynecol. Reprod. Biol. 2013.

78. de Punder K, Pruimboom L. The Dietary Intake of Wheat and other Cereal Grains and Their Role in Inflammation. Nutrients. 2013;5(3):771-787.

79. Biesiekierski JR, Newnham ED, Irving PM, et al. Gluten causes gastrointestinal symptoms in subjects without celiac disease: a double-blind randomized placebo-controlled trial. Am J Gastroenterol. 2011;106(3):508-514; quiz 515.

80. Ayyad C, Andersen T. Long-term efficacy of dietary treatment of obesity: a systematic review of studies published between 1931 and 1999. Obes Rev. 2000;1(2):113-119.

81. Bowen J, Noakes M, Clifton PM. A high dairy protein, high-calcium diet minimizes bone turnover in overweight adults during weight loss. J Nutr. 2004;134(3):568-573.

82. Ebbeling CB, Swain JF, Feldman HA, et al. Effects of dietary composition on energy expenditure during weight-loss maintenance. JAMA. 2012;307(24):2627-2634.

83. Luscombe-Marsh ND, Noakes M, Wittert GA, Keogh JB, Foster P, Clifton PM. Carbohydrate-restricted diets high in either monounsaturated fat or protein are equally effective at promoting fat loss and improving blood lipids. Am J Clin Nutr. 2005;81(4):762-772.

84. Altieri P, Cavazza C, Pasqui F, Morselli AM, Gambineri A, Pasquali R. Dietary habits and their relationship with hormones and metabolism in overweight and obese women with polycystic ovary syndrome. Clin Endocrinol. 2012.

85. Douglas CC, Norris LE, Oster RA, Darnell BE, Azziz R, Gower BA. Difference in dietary intake between women with polycystic ovary syndrome and healthy controls. Fertil Steril. 2006;86(2):411-417.

86. Meier U, Gressner AM. Endocrine regulation of energy metabolism: review of pathobiochemical and clinical chemical aspects of leptin, ghrelin, adiponectin, and resistin. Clin Chem. 2004;50(9):1511-1525.

87. English PJ, Ghatei MA, Malik IA, Bloom SR, Wilding JP. Food fails to suppress ghrelin levels in obese humans. J Clin Endocrinol Metab. 2002;87(6):2984.

88. Hosoda H, Kojima M, Kangawa K. Biological, physiological, and pharmacological aspects of ghrelin. J Pharmacol Sci. 2006;100(5):398-410.

89. Moran LJ, Noakes M, Clifton PM, et al. Postprandial ghrelin, cholecystokinin, peptide YY, and appetite before and after weight loss in

overweight women with and without polycystic ovary syndrome. Am J Clin Nutr. 2007;86(6):1603-1610.

90. Hirschberg AL, Naessen S, Stridsberg M, Bystrom B, Holtet J. Impaired cholecystokinin secretion and disturbed appetite regulation in women with polycystic ovary syndrome. Gynecol Endocrinol. 2004;19(2):79-87.

91. Golbahar J, Das NM, Al-Ayadhi MA, Gumaa K. Leptin-to-adiponectin, adiponectin-to-leptin ratios, and insulin are specific and sensitive markers associated with polycystic ovary syndrome: a case-control study from Bahrain. Metab Syndr Relat Disord. 2012;10(2):98-102.

92. Kedikova SE, Sirakov MM, Boyadzhieva MV. Leptin levels and adipose tissue percentage in adolescents with polycystic ovary syndrome. Gynecol Endocrinol. 2013;29(4):384-387.

93. Anderson JW, Konz EC, Frederich RC, Wood CL. Long-term weight-loss maintenance: a meta-analysis of US studies. Am J Clin Nutr. 2001;74(5): 579-584.

94. Jakicic JM, Otto AD. Treatment and prevention of obesity: what is the role of exercise? Nutr Rev. 2006;64(2 Pt 2):S57-61.

95. Penedo FJ, Dahn JR. Exercise and well-being: a review of mental and physical health benefits associated with physical activity. Curr Opin Psychiatry. 2005;18(2):189-193.

96. Americans DGf. 2008 Physical Activity Guidelines for Americans. 2008.

97. Norman RJ, Homan G, Moran L, Noakes M. Lifestyle choices, diet, and insulin sensitizers in polycystic ovary syndrome. Endocrine. 2006;30(1):35-43.

98. Moran LJ, Harrison CL, Hutchison SK, Stepto NK, Strauss BJ, Teede HJ. Exercise decreases anti-mullerian hormone in anovulatory overweight women with polycystic ovary syndrome: a pilot study. Horm Metab Res. 2011;43(13):977-979.

99. Palomba S, Giallauria F, Falbo A, et al. Structured exercise training programme versus hypocaloric hyperproteic diet in obese polycystic ovary syndrome patients with anovulatory infertility: a 24-week pilot study. Hum Reprod. 2008;23(3):642-650.

100.Brown AJ, Setji TL, Sanders LL, et al. Effects of exercise on lipoprotein particles in women with polycystic ovary syndrome. Med Sci Sports Exerc. 2009;41(3):497-504.

101.Cuff DJ, Meneilly GS, Martin A, Ignaszewski A, Tildesley HD, Frohlich JJ. Effective exercise modality to reduce insulin resistance in women with type 2 diabetes. Diabetes Care. 2003;26(11):2977-2982.

102.Kogure GS, Piccki FK, Vieira CS, Martins Wde P, dos Reis RM. Analysis of muscle strength and body composition of women with polycystic ovary syndrome. Rev Bras Ginecol Obstet. 2012;34(7):316-322.

103.Bruner B, Chad K, Chizen D. Effects of exercise and nutritional counseling in women with polycystic ovary syndrome. Appl Physiol Nutr Metab. 2006;31(4):384-391.

Chapter 3

ALTERNATIVE AND COMPLEMENTARY TREATMENTS

THE USE OF DIETARY AND HERBAL SUPPLEMENTS IN TREATING PCOS

Today, more and more people in the United States are turning to alternative treatments and complementary medicine to improve their health. According to the *Nutrition Business Journal*, U.S. consumers spent $30 billion on dietary supplements in 2011.[1] The trend is driven by several factors, including the increased availability of supplements, the desire to control personal health, the perception of increased safety, and disillusionment with traditional medicine. Women with PCOS who have not seen improvements in their symptoms generally grow frustrated with their medical care, so it's not surprising for them to turn to alternative treatments in hopes of getting better results.

There are always concerns with using alternative therapies, including supplement-medication interactions. This is particularly important considering that individuals do not always tell their physicians they are taking a dietary or herbal supplement. Many supplements and prescription or over-the-counter drugs utilize the same metabolic pathway in the liver, increasing the chances for an interaction that could alter how the supplement or medication works in the body, resulting in potentially harmful side effects or even death. For instance, increased vitamin K intake can affect the action of the oral anticoagulant warfarin (Coumadin), leading to blood clots. Similarly, the antiandrogen medication spironolactone is a potassium-sparing diuretic, so taking potassium supplements in addition to spironolactone could cause dangerously high blood levels of potassium, possibly resulting in heart failure and death.

Another major concern is supplement safety. The FDA does not monitor dietary supplements as closely as it does food or drugs, nor does it determine whether products are safe before they go to market. The FDA Good Manufacturing Practices, a set of recommendations and expectations, ensures the identity, purity, strength, and composition of dietary supplements so that they are processed in a consistent manner and meet quality standards. By law, manufacturers are required to report adverse dietary supplement events to the FDA.

Many people may think there's no harm in taking supplements because they are "natural" or "safe." This may cause people to exceed the recommended dosage or combine supplements with other supplements or medications in the hopes of improving their effectiveness.

Many women with PCOS take metformin, which helps reduce blood glucose. Numerous dietary and herbal supplements can also reduce glucose, increasing the risk of hypoglycemia. Therefore, it is important to properly screen women with PCOS for supplement use and inform clients of any potential risk.

Compliance is an important factor. For optimal effectiveness, supplements should be taken daily. However, sporadic adherence is not uncommon when someone is taking multiple supplements and medications at different intervals throughout the day. Dietitians and other health care professionals can assist with establishing a routine to increase supplement compliance.

In light of their increasing popularity and because some demonstrate positive results for women with PCOS, dietitians should familiarize themselves with herbal and dietary supplements. The following are some effective and common supplements used among women with PCOS as an alternative or adjunct to their current medical treatment. The benefits of acupuncture and other alternative treatments are also discussed.

N-Acetylcysteine
Purported use: insulin resistance, infertility, androgen lowering, dyslipidemia
Recommended dosage: 1.6 to 3 g/day

N-acetylcystine (NAC) is both an antioxidant and amino acid. Specifically, it's a derivative of the amino acid L-cysteine, an essential precursor used by the body to produce glutathione, an antioxidant that protects against free radical damage and is a critical factor in supporting a healthy immune system. NAC has numerous uses, from treating bronchitis to removing heavy metals and environmental pollutants from the body. It's also been found to reduce inflammation, total and LDL cholesterol, and, most recently, insulin.

A study published in the *European Journal of Obstetrics, Gynecology, and Reproductive Biology* compared the effects of NAC and metformin.[2] In this prospective trial, 100 women with PCOS were divided to receive either metformin (500 mg three times daily) or NAC (600 mg three times daily) for 24 weeks. Both treatments resulted in significant and equal decreases in BMI, hirsutism, fasting insulin, free testosterone, and menstrual irregularity. NAC led to a significant decrease in both total and LDL cholesterol, whereas metformin led to only a decrease in total cholesterol.

This research supports findings published in the *Journal of Fertility and Sterility*, where researchers reported significant improvements in insulin sensitivity after five weeks among women with PCOS who took 1.6 to 3 g/day of NAC and had elevated insulin levels before the start of study.[3] Women treated with NAC showed significant improvements in testosterone, cholesterol, and TG levels.[3]

In regard to fertility, three randomized studies compared NAC or metformin with Clomid in PCOS.[4-6] In two of the studies, Clomid plus NAC resulted in improved ovulation and pregnancy rates compared with placebo.[4,6] However, this group experienced fewer instances of ovulation and pregnancy when compared with metformin and Clomid.[5]

Overall, NAC is well tolerated but can cause adverse GI effects, including nausea, abdominal pain, vomiting, constipation, and diarrhea, particularly when used in high doses. Based on the related studies, the therapeutic dosage of NAC to improve insulin sensitivity is 1.6 to 3 g/day, not to exceed 8 g/day.[7] Women who are overweight or obese may benefit from a higher dose. Fulghesu et al[3] found that patients with PCOS who were obese did not respond to doses of NAC under 3 g/day.

Since NAC oxidizes quickly, an effervescent tablet is recommended over pill form.[7]

Alpha-Lipoic Acid
Purported use: diabetes, insulin resistance
Recommended dosage: 300 to 1,200 mg/day

Alpha-lipoic acid (ALA) is synthesized in the mitochondria and is a potent antioxidant. It is involved in carbohydrate metabolism and has been shown to improve blood glucose, insulin sensitivity,[8,9] and neuropathy in T2DM.[10]

Studies involving the use of ALA in PCOS are scarce. Six lean women with PCOS who took 1,200 mg of controlled-release ALA daily for 16 weeks experienced a 13.5% improvement in insulin sensitivity; triglyceride levels also improved.[11] Doses up to 2,000 mg/day have been well tolerated; however, ALA should be used with caution as some side effects, including skin reactions, GI upset, and possible hypoglycemia, have been reported with high dosages.[12]

Red meat, yeast, liver, kidney, spinach, broccoli, and potatoes are good sources of ALA.

Bitter Melon or Bitter Gourd (*Momordica charantia*)

Purported use: diabetes, hypoglycemic agent
Recommended dosage: 50 to 100 mL (3 to 6 T)/day

Bitter melon, a vegetable grown in tropical countries worldwide, has been used as a traditional herbal medicine and food for thousands of years.[13] It is best known for lowering blood glucose in people with diabetes, as it may mimic insulin.[14]

A Cochrane review of two RCTs found no significant difference in glycemic control with bitter melon compared with placebo or metformin.[15] However, bitter melon was found to improve metabolic syndrome and waist circumference in a small sample of men and women.[16]

Bitter melon may increase the risk of hypoglycemia, as it can have additive effects on blood sugar when used with other supplements or medications. Hypoglycemic coma, convulsions in children, and reduced fertility in mice have been documented.[14]

Bitter melon is sold as a tea or in capsule form.

Chasteberry (*Vitex agnus-castus*)

Purported use: acne, infertility, hormone regulation,
menstrual irregularities, PMS
Recommended dosage: 20 to 40 mg/day

Chasteberry is an herb used for centuries for its role in regulating hormone levels and menstrual and fertility disorders. Preliminary evidence suggests that chasteberry may have phytoestrogen effects.[17] This herb is proposed to stimulate the pituitary gland and increase levels of LH and progesterone, increasing the chance of pregnancy.

A double-blind, placebo-controlled pilot study examined the effects on fertility of a nutritional supplement containing chasteberry, green tea extracts, L-arginine, vitamins and minerals in which five of the 15 women (33%) in the treatment group became pregnant after three months of use.[18] Women who took the nutritional supplement had increased midluteal progesterone levels.

Chasteberry does not work quickly and may take three to seven months to promote pregnancy.[17] It should not be taken by women who already are pregnant.

Chasteberry is generally well tolerated. Side effects may include GI complaints, dizziness, headache, lethargy, and dry mouth.[17,19] It may interfere with dopamine-antagonist medications (eg, Zyprexa, Risperdal).[17]

Chromium Picolinate

Purported use: diabetes, insulin resistance
Recommended dosage: 500 to 1,000 mcg/day

Chromium is an essential trace mineral involved in carbohydrate metabolism and known for its role in potentiating insulin.[20] A chromium deficiency is associated with impaired glucose, insulin, and lipid metabolism.[20] Chromium supplementation may be effective in lowering glucose and insulin levels in people with diabetes and insulin resistance.[21-23]

A review of 15 studies on chromium supplementation showed that chromium deficiency results in insulin resistance.[23] Another conclusion was that insulin resistance caused by chromium deficiency can be improved with supplementation.[23] However, a randomized, double-blind, placebo-controlled trial found that treatment with 400 mcg/day for six months did not improve glycemic control in people with diabetes.[24]

A small study involving five obese women with PCOS and insulin resistance demonstrated encouraging results with chromium supplementation. The women took 1,000 mcg/day for two months without changing their diet or activity level and experienced a 38% improvement in glucose.[25]

Another small pilot study found that 200 mcg/day improved glucose tolerance in women with PCOS. No affect was found in regard to ovulatory function or hormonal parameters.[26] To validate these results, well-controlled randomized trials will need to be conducted.

Rich food sources include brewer's yeast, intact whole grains, mushrooms, broccoli, dried beans, and seeds. Generally, chromium is well tolerated. Side effects may include headaches, insomnia, sleep disturbances, irritability, and mood changes.[20] Chromium may cause hypoglycemia in patients taking medications to treat diabetes.

Rich food sources include brewer's yeast, intact whole grains, mushrooms, broccoli, dried beans, and seeds.

Cinnamon Cassia
Purported use: insulin resistance, diabetes, dyslipidemia
Recommended dosage: 1 to 6 g/day

Cinnamon is a popular spice believed to increase the phosphorylation of insulin receptors, which leads to improved insulin function and insulin sensitivity.[27] It may also reduce postprandial insulin response by delaying gastric emptying.[28]

A meta-analysis of six RCTs showed that cinnamon resulted in significant decreases in HbA1c and fasting plasma glucose in people with T2DM.[29]

Another trial reported that cassia cinnamon lowered total cholesterol, LDL cholesterol, and triglycerides in T2DM.[30] Fifteen women with PCOS were randomized to take cinnamon or a placebo for eight weeks. The cinnamon group experienced significant reductions in insulin resistance.[27]

Since it may lower glucose and insulin levels, it's important to carefully monitor blood sugar levels to prevent hypoglycemia. Cinnamon has not been shown to cause any adverse effects.[31]

This tasty spice can be sprinkled on foods such as cereal, applesauce, peanut butter sandwiches, oatmeal, and coffee or taken in capsule form. One teaspoon of ground cinnamon equals 3 g.

Fenugreek (Trigonella foenum-graecum)

Purported use: increase milk production
and breast growth, diabetes, insulin resistance
Recommended dosage: 10 to 15 g/day

Fenugreek is a popular and effective herbal supplement used by nursing mothers to boost milk supply. It may help with breast development, which is a cause of insufficient milk production in PCOS. It is also sold in teas known as Mother's Milk, which contains fennel and other herbs used to boost milk production.

There are no apparent side effects in babies whose mothers take fenugreek. Most mothers will see an increase in milk supply within 24 to 72 hours.[32] Pregnant women should not take fenugreek, as it may stimulate the uterus, causing contractions.[33]

Fenugreek has been shown to reduce glucose and insulin levels.[34-37] In a double-blind placebo-controlled study of 25 individuals with T2DM, fenugreek improved glycemic control, insulin resistance, and triglycerides.[37] Fenugreek seeds contain 50% dietary fiber and pectin, and may affect GI transit, slowing glucose absorption.[33,36]

People with diabetes should use this seed with caution, as it may cause hypoglycemia.[33] Additionally, fenugreek may have antiplatelet activity and should be used with caution when taking anticoagulants.[33] Possible side effects of fenugreek include gas, bloating, and diarrhea.

Fenugreek seeds can be eaten whole, sprouted, or ground into a spice or flour used in baking.

Garlic

Purported use: dyslipidemia, hypertension, menstrual disorders
Recommended dosage: Fresh garlic 4 grams/day (approximately one clove)
or Garlic extract 600-1200 mg

Garlic is a bulb from the Liliaceae plant family that has been used both as a medicine and a spice for thousands of years. Garlic's most common uses are for high cholesterol, heart disease, hypertension, and menstrual disorders.

Preliminary research suggests that taking garlic may slow the development of atherosclerosis. A meta-analysis of 26 studies showed garlic could reduce total cholesterol and triglyceride levels; no influence on LDL and HDL levels were shown.[38]

Garlic is well tolerated but can thin the blood in a manner similar to aspirin. It should be used with caution if surgery or dental work is needed or in people with bleeding disorders.[39]

Gymnema sylvestre
Purposed use: diabetes, insulin resistance, dyslipidemia
Recommended dosage: 400 to 600 mg/day

Gymnema sylvestre, also known as gurmar ("sugar destroyer" in Hindi), is a traditional Ayurvedic herb used as an antidiabetic, hypoglycemic agent.[40] It is believed that gymnema stimulates insulin release from the pancreas.[41]

In one study, 400 mg/day was given to 22 patients with T2DM for 18 to 20 months, with the result being significant reductions in blood glucose and HbA1c. Five patients maintained blood sugar control with gymnema without the help of oral medication.[42] To date, however, no studies have examined gymnema use in PCOS.

Side-effects include taste alteration and hypoglycemia.[43]

Inositol (D-chiro-inositol and Myo-inositol)
Purposed use: insulin resistance, dyslipidemia, androgen lowering, infertility, hypertension, weight loss
Recommended dosage: 1.2 to 4 g/day

Myo-inositol (MYO) and D-chiro-inositol (DCI) are perhaps the most researched nutritional supplements for PCOS. Relatives of the B complex vitamins, MYO and DCI have shown favorable results in improving nearly all aspects of PCOS, including insulin sensitivity,[44,45] reproduction (MYO restores ovulation and improves oocyte quality),[46-50] hormonal imbalance, (improves androgens)[44] and metabolic issues (inflammation, dyslipidemia, hypertension, and weight loss).[45,50,51] Because of the many benefits, MYO and DCI are important supplements that should be considered as part of the first-line treatment for PCOS.

MYO and DCI act as inositol-phosphoglycan (IPG) mediators, or secondary messengers, relaying signals from insulin receptors on the cell membrane to the cell nucleus.[49] It is believed that women with PCOS have a defect in the insulin-signaling pathway as well as altered metabolism of inositol, which may contribute to insulin resistance.[49,52,53]

Glucose inhibits inositol;[54] individuals with T2DM have been shown to have reduced levels of DCI.[55,56] Metformin has been shown to improve the action of insulin by improving DCI IPG mediators.[57]

Inositol improves metabolic factors in PCOS. A large randomized, double-blind, placebo-controlled trial showed that MYO (4 g/day) increased HDL levels and resulted in significant weight loss in women with PCOS, although no change in insulin was detected.[50] Another double-blind placebo trial showed that MYO (4 g/day) decreased insulin, triglycerides, testosterone, and blood pressure in women with PCOS.[45]

More recently, Venturella et al showed that 2 g/day of MYO for six months resulted in significant weight loss and improved HDL and LDL levels.[48] MYO at 1,200 mg/day for 12 weeks significantly decreased androgens and insulin in non-obese women with PCOS.[44]

It has been suggested that MYO can prevent GDM in women with PCOS. The prevalence of GDM in the MYO group was 17.4% compared with 54% in the control group.[58]

While MYO and DCI have similar actions, they are different molecules (MYO converts into DCI) and are believed to regulate different biological processes.[59] Combined administration of MYO and DCI was shown to be more effective in improving metabolic parameters in overweight women with PCOS compared with MYO alone.[59]

In regard to fertility, MYO improved oocyte quality better than DCI, as shown in a randomized trial.[46] MYO has also been demonstrated to restore ovulation.[50] Twenty-two of 25 women with PCOS had restored menstrual cycle with six months of MYO treatment; 72% of them maintained normal ovulation, and 40% became pregnant.[60]

Raffone et al compared the effects of metformin and MYO in women with PCOS.[61] Sixty women received 1,500 mg/day of metformin, while 60 women received 4 g/day of MYO plus 400 mcg of folic acid. Ovulation was restored in 65% of women treated with MYO vs. 50% in the metformin group. More pregnancies occurred in the MYO group vs. metformin (18% vs. 11%).[61]

DCI also improved ovulation. Women with PCOS who were given 1,200 mg of DCI for six to eight weeks had an ovulation rate of 86% vs. only 27% in those who received a placebo.[51]

MYO at doses of 2 to 4 g was was well tolerated in women with PCOS with no reported side effects.[62] Hypoglycemia and mild GI side effects such as nausea, flatus, and diarrhea occurred at 12 g/

day.[63] Since it may lower glucose and insulin levels, it's important to carefully monitor blood sugar levels to prevent hypoglycemia.

Maca (Lepidium meyenii)
Purported use: hypoglycemic, cholesterol, hormone regulation, infertility, anemia
Recommended dosage: 1.5 to 3 g/day

Maca, a member of the radish family that is rich in iron and contains polyunsaturated fats, is exclusively grown in the Andes mountains of Peru and known for its role in treating anemia, infertility, and female hormone balance.[64] At least 13 different types of maca are grown.

A member of the radish family, maca is iron-rich and contains polyunsaturated fats. A systematic review of four RCTs found that maca had favorable effects on menopausal symptoms in healthy, early, and late postmenopausal women.[64]

Maca appears to be safe in doses up to 3 g/day for 12 weeks.[65] It can be used as flour in baking or added to smoothies or other beverages and food or taken in capsule form.

Magnesium
Purported use: diabetes, insulin resistance, hypertension, osteoporosis
Recommended dosage: 600 to 1,000 mg/day

Magnesium is an essential mineral important in bone structure, fat and protein synthesis, and carbohydrate metabolism, and is involved in more than 300 different enzyme systems. Magnesium supplementation may be beneficial for women with PCOS because of its ability to reduce insulin, glucose, lipids, and blood pressure.[66-69]

A higher intake of magnesium is associated with a 31% lower risk of young adults developing metabolic syndrome.[68] Magnesium helps regulate glucose levels by influencing the release and activity of insulin.[70,71] The Women's Health Study showed an inverse association between magnesium intake and the risk of T2DM, independent of age and BMI.[72]

Sharifi et al[73] found the risk of PCOS for women with magnesium deficiency was 19 times greater than for those who had normal magnesium concentrations. No correlation was found between magnesium and insulin sensitivity or secretion, glucose, lipids, and androgen concentrations. The authors suggested that women with PCOS may have low magnesium levels secondary to calcium and vitamin D deficiency, and that serum calcium levels are a better predictor of PCOS than magnesium.[73] Muneyyirci et al also found significantly lower magnesium in PCOS patients compared with controls.

However, Kauffman et al did not find hypomagnesemia among women with PCOS and concluded that magnesium levels did not correspond with age, BMI, waist circumference, insulin sensitivity, glycemic levels, blood pressure, or lipid levels in a small sample of reproductive-age women with PCOS.[74]

Magnesium is found in certain types of fish, whole grains, fruits, nuts, green vegetables seeds, and legumes.[66] It can cause GI irritation, nausea, vomiting, and diarrhea. Although rare, large amounts may cause hypermagnesemia with symptoms including thirst, hypotension, drowsiness, confusion, muscle weakness, cardiac arrhythmias, coma, cardiac arrest, and death.[75] High doses of zinc (greater than 142 mg/day) can decrease magnesium absorption as zinc and magnesium compete for transport in the body. Magnesium also can affect the absorption of antibiotics.[75]

Milk Thistle (Silybum marianum)
Purported use: liver disease, cholesterol, anti-inflammatory, insulin resistance, galactagogue, antioxidant
Recommended dosage: 200 to 600 mg/day

Milk thistle extracts have been used as a "liver tonic" for centuries and may benefit women with PCOS who have fatty liver disease or elevated liver enzymes. Milk thistle has been shown to improve liver disease and protect against hepatic toxins, and also has resulted in decreased hepatic inflammation and fibrosis.[76] It also may improve glycemic control in T2DM.[76,77] However, there are no known studies of milk thistle in PCOS.

Taking 200 mg three times per day for four months, in combination with conventional treatment, significantly decreased fasting blood glucose, HbA1c, total cholesterol, LDL cholesterol, and triglycerides compared with placebo in patients with T2DM.[78] Milk thistle also may increase milk supply in lactating mothers.[79]

Milk thistle seeds can be eaten raw or toasted or they can be ground into a powder to add to food. It can also be taken in capsule form. Milk thistle does not show significant interactions with other drugs.[76] Side effects may include nausea, diarrhea, dyspepsia, flatulence, and abdominal bloating.

Omega-3 Fatty Acids
Purported use: anti-inflammatory, dyslipidemia, hypertension, depression, androgen lowering, infertility, insulin resistance, liver disease
Recommended dosage: up to 4 g/day

Omega-3 PUFAs, specifically long-chain eicosapentaenoic acid (EPA) and docosahexaenoic acid (DHA) found in cold-water fish, offer numerous health benefits to women with PCOS, including increased insulin sensitivity; reduced hyperinsulinemia; lowered plasma triglycerides, liver fat, and androgens; decreased inflammation, and improved symptoms of depression.[80-85] The plant-derived short-chain omega-3, alpha-linolenic acid (ALA) is slowly converted into EPA and DHA.

Omega-3 PUFAs metabolically compete for absorption with omega-6 PUFAs so that a diet rich in omega-6 fats (the typical Western diet) may be deficient in omega-3 fats. One study showed that ALA intake is inversely associated with metabolic syndrome.[86] Despite its metabolic benefits, a meta-analysis involving 20 studies concluded omega-3 PUFA supplementation was not associated with a lower risk of all-cause mortality, cardiac death, sudden death, myocardial infarction, or stroke.[87]

Omega-3 fats may be effective in improving insulin resistance, BMI, and hirsutism in women with PCOS. Forty-five nonobese women with PCOS were given 1,500mg of omega-3 for six months. Reductions in BMI and insulin levels were found along with improvements in LH, testosterone, and SHBG levels.[85]

A double-blind RCT showed that treatment with 4 g/day of fish oil for eight weeks significantly reduced glucose, insulin, triglycerides, and LDL cholesterol and increased HDL cholesterol in women with PCOS who were overweight or obese.[88] In their respective RCTs, Cussons et al and Vargas et al also showed fish oil decreased triglyceride levels in women with PCOS, but no improvement in insulin sensitivity, total cholesterol, and LDL and

HDL levels were found.[89,90] Additionally, neither of the studies showed improvements in anthropometric measurements or CRP levels.

These studies showed mixed effects with omega-3 supplementation and improvement of insulin resistance in PCOS. A meta-analysis of 11 RCTs showed omega-3 PUFAs have no effect on insulin sensitivity in women without PCOS.[91]

Omega-3 fats may help with fertility.[92,93] Female androgen concentrations were significantly reduced after supplementation of long-chain omega-3 fats.[82] In contrast, omega-6 PUFAs have been shown to inhibit embryo maturation.[93]

Patients should be advised about ways to regularly incorporate foods rich in omega-3 PUFAs into their diet, such as including at least two 3.5-oz servings of fatty types of fish each week or taking fish oil supplements regularly. Fish oil supplements are generally well tolerated but may cause heartburn, nausea, and loose stools in some individuals; taking them with food may decrease these side effects. The FDA has concluded that up to 4 g of EPA and DHA is generally recognized as safe. Fish oil doses greater than 4 g/day or a high dietary intake of fish (greater than 46 g/day) may inhibit platelet aggregation and cause bleeding.[94]

More information on the role of omega-3 fats in treating PCOS is located in Chapter 2.

Prickly Pear Cactus (Opunita ficus-indica)
Purported use: insulin resistance
Recommended dosage: 100 to 500 g/day

The stems of the prickly pear cactus fruit have traditionally been used in Mexico to treat T2DM. However, most evidence is based in animal models. It is believed the high fibrous pectin content of prickly pear cactus can slow carbohydrate absorption and decrease lipid absorption from the gut.[95]

An RCT involving a natural fiber complex (Litramine IQP) derived from prickly pear cactus showed significantly reduced BMI, body fat composition, and waist circumference in humans.[96]

Side effects include mild diarrhea, nausea, abdominal fullness, and headache.[95] It also has additive effects with diabetes medications and potentially cause hypoglycemia.

The sweet, mineral-rich fruit can be eaten whole or made into juice.

St. John's Wort (Hypericum perforatum)
Purported use: mild to moderate depression
Recommended dosage: 300 to 1,200 mg/day

St. John's wort, the most widely used antidepressant in Germany, is a plant known for its use in treating mild to moderate depression. It is a selective inhibitor of serotonin, dopamine, and norepinephrine reuptake in the central nervous system, much like prescribed antidepressants.[97]

A meta-analysis of 29 studies concluded St. John's wort was superior to placebo in patients with major depression and is similarly effective as standard antidepressants with fewer side effects.[98]

Overall, it is well tolerated. Adverse effects include photosensitization, headache, nausea, abdominal discomfort, and dry mouth.[99] Because St. John's wort is metabolized in the liver by the cytochrome P450 system, it can increase or decrease the elimination of many prescription drugs or herbs. It also may decrease the effectiveness of birth control medications.

St. John's wort should not be taken with other herbal supplements, antidepressants, or mood stabilizers and is contraindicated in pregnancy.[99]

Saw Palmetto (Serenoa repens)
Purported use: androgen lowering, anti-inflammatory
Recommended dosage: 160 to 320 mg/day

Native to North America, saw palmetto is a popular herbal supplement among women with PCOS because of its proposed antiandrogenic effects. The berries of the saw palmetto palm contain sterols, fatty acids, and flavonoids believed to inhibit the enzyme 5 alpha-reductase that converts testosterone to dihydrotestosterone, a hormone that stimulates hirsutism in women with PCOS. One study showed obese and normal-weight women with PCOS had higher levels of 5 alpha-reductase.[100]

To date, no studies have examined the effects of saw palmetto in PCOS. However, an RCT showed saw palmetto was effective in the treatment of androgenic alopecia in men.[101] It is unknown whether saw palmetto may help women with PCOS who suffer from androgenic alopecia.

No adverse effects or herb-drug interactions have been reported.[102] Side effects are minor and include dizziness, headaches, and GI disturbances.[102] Patients may need to take saw palmetto for six weeks to see noticeable changes.[102] It should not be used while taking OCPs because it can alter hormone levels.[102]

Vitamin D

Purported use: insulin resistance, diabetes, infertility, dyslipidemia
Recommended dosage: 1,500 to 2,000 IU/day

Vitamin D deficiency has become an epidemic in the United States.[103] A deficiency of vitamin D not only causes poor bone mineralization but also has been implicated in numerous chronic diseases, including diabetes, metabolic syndrome, heart disease, cancer, and hypertension.[103-105]

Low vitamin D status is highly prevalent among the PCOS population.[106,107] Studies examining vitamin D status in women with PCOS showed an inverse relationship between vitamin D and metabolic risk factors (insulin resistance, BMI, triglycerides, HDL cholesterol).[106,108] Lower levels of vitamin D have been shown in women with PCOS who are obese compared with those who aren't obese.[106]

Vitamin D, a hormone, is involved in insulin action. It is unclear whether vitamin D insufficiency is a result of obesity or whether obesity is a cause of vitamin D insufficiency.[106] A RCT failed to show the effect of vitamin D supplementation on insulin sensitivity and insulin resistance in women with PCOS.[109] More RCTs to determine the effectiveness of vitamin D on insulin resistance are needed.

Vitamin D affects reproduction, as it has been shown to be involved in follicle egg maturation and development.[110] Supplementation with vitamin D may improve ovulation and conception in women with PCOS.[107,110,111] In a small trial of 13 women with PCOS who were vitamin D deficient, normal menstrual cycles resumed within two months in seven women when given vitamin D repletion with calcium therapy.[110] The study authors suggest that abnormalities in calcium homeostasis may be responsible for the arrested follicular development in women with PCOS.[110]

Other studies have shown the benefits of vitamin D in improving infertility treatments in women with PCOS.[112] Vitamin D deficiency also is common in pregnant women.[111] Low vitamin D is linked with GDM and preeclampsia.[113]

The optimal amount of vitamin D for women with PCOS is unknown. The DRI for vitamin D is 600 IU/day, but this may not be sufficient for women with PCOS. The Tolerable Upper Limit for vitamin D is 4,000 IU/day; however, no adverse effects have been found with up to 10,000 IU/day.[114]

Few foods contain vitamin D other than milk fortified with vitamin D, eggs, cereals with vitamin D added, and fatty fish. While skin exposure to the sun provides as much as 80% to 90% of the body's vitamin D, production is limited with sunscreen use and based on geographic location.

Blood levels of vitamin D can be measured by serum 25-hydroxyvitamin D (25(OH)D). Vitamin D deficiency is defined as 25(OH)D below 20 ng/mL.[115] The Endocrine Practice Committee has suggested a vitamin D intake of 1,500 to 2000 IU/day to maintain a blood level of 25(OH)D consistently above 30 ng/mL.[115] The committee also suggested that adults who are vitamin D deficient be treated with 50,000 IU of vitamin D2 or D3 once per week for eight weeks (or its equivalent of 6,000 IU/day) to achieve a 25(OH)D level above 30 ng/mL.[115]

Vitamin B12

Purported use: deficiency prevention with metformin
and oral contraceptive pill use
Recommended dosage: 500 to 1,000 mcg/daily; Recommended Dietary
Allowance: 2.4 mcg/day

Vitamin B12 is a water-soluble vitamin required for proper red blood cell formation, neurological function, and DNA synthesis. As a cofactor in the conversion of homocysteine to methionine, B12 plays a role in heart disease prevention.[116] It is found primarily in foods such as beef, fish, eggs, and dairy products. Individuals who follow a vegan diet are at risk of B12 deficiency.

It has been proposed that low serum B12 may be a marker of possible adiposity and insulin resistance in women with PCOS.[117] Low vitamin B12 concentrations were shown in women with PCOS who were obese and had insulin resistance compared with women with PCOS but no insulin resistance and non-PCOS weight-matched controls. Treatment with B12 improved insulin resistance in patients with metabolic syndrome.[118]

Metformin use causes malabsorption of vitamin B12, possibly through increased bacterial overgrowth or alterations of the vitamin B12-intrinsic factor complex or intestinal mobility.[116] Thus, metformin therapy may increase homocysteine levels.[119] Kilicdag et al[119] observed a 19.78% decrease in vitamin B12 levels in women with PCOS treated with metformin for three months. Women with PCOS tend to take high amounts of metformin; long-term use at high doses is a risk factor for vitamin B12 deficiency.[117] Mandatory B12 supplementation has been proposed for those taking metformin.[120]

In addition to metformin, oral contraceptive pills (OCPs) which are commonly prescribed for PCOS, have been shown to decrease vitamin B12 levels.[121]

Symptoms of vitamin B12 deficiency include certain types of anemia, infertility, neuropathy, chronic fatigue, memory loss, confusion, and depression. Individuals who take metformin should have their vitamin B12 levels checked annually. A blood test can assess vitamin B12 status, with the optimal level being greater than 450 pg/mL.[116] Elevated serum homocysteine and urinary methylmalonic acid levels, the gold standard in assessing B12, also indicate deficiency.

COMPLEMENTARY TREATMENTS FOR PCOS

Acupuncture

Acupuncture, a form of traditional Chinese medicine that dates back more than 3,000 years, may be beneficial for restoring ovulation, treating menstrual disturbances, and improving metabolic function in women with PCOS.[122,123] This drug-free philosophy is based on restoring chi, or energy flow, within the body.

There are believed to be more than 2,000 acupuncture points in the body. A blockage of energy at one of these points is thought to be the cause of an illness, pain, or injury.

"Acupuncture therapy may have a role in PCOS by increasing of blood flow to the ovaries, reducing of ovarian volume and the number of ovarian cysts, controlling hyperglycemia through increasing insulin sensitivity and decreasing blood glucose and insulin levels, reducing cortisol levels and assisting in weight loss."[124]

Many nonrandomized studies have been conducted documenting the success of acupuncture in improving PCOS; however, few RCTs have been done. In one study, 24 women with PCOS who had irregular periods underwent electroacupuncture, a form of acupuncture that stimulates electric currents through the needles. After 10 to 14 treatments, 38% of the women experienced regular ovulation.[122] A meta-analysis of 17 studies concluded acupuncture did not significantly improve in vitro fertilization or intracytoplasmic sperm injection.[125]

Other Complementary Treatments

In addition to acupuncture, other forms of complementary treatments may be beneficial in treating PCOS. Acupressure, reflexology, Reiki, mindfulness, and aromatherapy are all treatments that may improve PCOS symptoms. Tai chi and yoga are forms of physical activity that have also been shown to be benefit women with PCOS.

In summary, dietary and herbal supplements are rising in popularity among Americans. Many women with PCOS who are frustrated with their symptoms and medical treatment may turn to alternative treatments instead of or in conjunction with medications to improve fertility and other symptoms. Therefore, dietitians need to familiarize themselves with these and other supplements common among the PCOS community.

Safety is a big concern, as dietary supplements are not well regulated by the FDA and clinical trials are limited in duration and sample size. The recommendation for any supplement should be individualized and given after completing a detailed nutrition assessment where diet intake and supplement (including multivitamins) and medication use are assessed, and the patient's metabolic risk factors and treatment goals have been considered. The dietitian must educate the patient on the benefits and risks of each supplement.

Once a supplement is recommended, careful monitoring by the dietitian, physician, and patient is necessary. Food supplements, such as garlic and cinnamon, can be encouraged as part of a healthy diet and are considered safe in the doses stated above. Other supplements discussed here have shown some efficacy in improving PCOS; however, there are side effects, and caution should be exhibited when using any of them. Hypoglycemia, for instance, is a common side effect in supplements that play a role in improving insulin sensitivity. Taking more than one supplement to improve insulin thus increases the risk for hypoglycemia. It is best to introduce one supplement at a time and monitor for side effects before recommending additional supplements.

Last, although dietary supplements may improve certain aspects of PCOS, they are not a substitute for lifestyle modification. Patients should always discuss supplement use with their physicians prior to use.

REFERENCES

1. NBJ's Supplement Business Report. Nutrition Business Journal;2012.
2. One r G, Muderris, II. Clinical, endocrine and metabolic effects of metformin vs N-acetyl-cysteine in women with polycystic ovary syndrome. Europ J obstet gynecol reprod biol. 2011;159(1):127-131.
3. Fulghesu AM, Ciampelli M, Muzj G, et al. N-acetyl-cysteine treatment improves insulin sensitivity in women with polycystic ovary syndrome. Fertil steril. 2002;77(6):1128-1135.
4. Salehpour S, Akbari Sene A, Saharkhiz N, Sohrabi MR, Moghimian F. N-acetylcysteine as an adjuvant to clomiphene citrate for successful induction of ovulation in infertile patients with polycystic ovary syndrome. J Obstet Gynaecol Res. 2012;38(9):1182-1186.
5. Abu Hashim H, Anwar K, El-Fatah RA. N-acetyl cysteine plus clomiphene citrate versus metformin and clomiphene citrate in treatment of clomiphene-resistant polycystic ovary syndrome: a randomized controlled trial. J Women's Health (2002). 2010;19(11):2043-2048.
6. Rizk AY, Bedaiwy MA, Al-Inany HG. N-acetyl-cysteine is a novel adjuvant to clomiphene citrate in clomiphene citrate-resistant patients with polycystic ovary syndrome. Fertil Steril. 2005;83(2):367-370.
7. Atkuri KR, Mantovani JJ, Herzenberg LA, Herzenberg LA. N-Acetylcysteine--a safe antidote for cysteine/glutathione deficiency. Current opinion in pharmacol. 2007;7(4):355-359.
8. Ansar H, Mazloom Z, Kazemi F, Hejazi N. Effect of alpha-lipoic acid on blood glucose, insulin resistance and glutathione peroxidase of type 2 diabetic patients. Saudi medical journal. 2011;32(6):584-588.
9. Jacob S, Ruus P, Hermann R, et al. Oral administration of RAC-alpha-lipoic acid modulates insulin sensitivity in patients with type-2 diabetes mellitus: a placebo-controlled pilot trial. Free Radic Biol Med. 1999;27(3-4):309-314.
10. Han T, Bai J, Liu W, Hu Y. A systematic review and meta-analysis of alpha-lipoic acid in the treatment of diabetic peripheral neuropathy. Europ J endocrinol. 2012;167(4):465-471.
11. Masharani U, Gjerde C, Evans JL, Youngren JF, Goldfine ID. Effects of controlled-release alpha lipoic acid in lean, nondiabetic patients with polycystic ovary syndrome. J diabetes sci technol. 2010;4(2):359-364.
12. Packer L, Tritschler HJ, Wessel K. Neuroprotection by the metabolic antioxidant alpha-lipoic acid. Free Radic Biol Med. 1997;22(1-2):359-378.
13. Singh J, Cumming E, Manoharan G, Kalasz H, Adeghate E. Medicinal chemistry

of the anti-diabetic effects of momordica charantia: active constituents and modes of actions. Open medicinal chemistry. 2011;5(Suppl 2):70-77.

14. Basch E, Gabardi S, Ulbricht C. Bitter melon (Momordica charantia): a review of efficacy and safety. American journal of health-system pharmacy. AJHP. 2003;60(4):356-359.

15. Ooi CP, Yassin Z, Hamid TA. Momordica charantia for type 2 diabetes mellitus. Cochrane Database Syst Rev. 2012;8:CD007845.

16. Tsai CH, Chen EC, Tsay HS, Huang CJ. Wild bitter gourd improves metabolic syndrome: a preliminary dietary supplementation trial. Nutrition journal. 2012;11:4.

17. Chasteberry. Natural Medicines Comprehensive Database. Accessed January 7, 2013.

18. Westphal LM, Polan ML, Trant AS, Mooney SB. A nutritional supplement for improving fertility in women: a pilot study. J Reprod Med. 2004;49(4):289-293.

19. Roemheld-Hamm B. Chasteberry. Amer family physician. 2005;72(5):821-824.

20. A scientific review: the role of chromium in insulin resistance. Diabetes educator. 2004;Suppl:2-14.

21. Vladeva SV, Terzieva DD, Arabadjiiska DT. Effect of chromium on the insulin resistance in patients with type II diabetes mellitus. Folia medica. 2005;47(3-4):59-62.

22. Anderson RA, Cheng N, Bryden NA, et al. Elevated intakes of supplemental chromium improve glucose and insulin variables in individuals with type 2 diabetes. Diabetes. 1997;46(11):1786-1791.

23. Mertz W. Chromium in human nutrition: a review. J Nutr. 1993;123(4):626-633.

24. Kleefstra N, Houweling ST, Bakker SJ, et al. Chromium treatment has no effect in patients with type 2 diabetes in a Western population: a randomized, double-blind, placebo-controlled trial. Diabetes Care. 2007;30(5):1092-1096.

25. Lydic ML, McNurlan M, Bembo S, Mitchell L, Komaroff E, Gelato M. Chromium picolinate improves insulin sensitivity in obese subjects with polycystic ovary syndrome. Fertil steril. 2006;86(1):243-246.

26. Lucidi RS, Thyer AC, Easton CA, Holden AE, Schenken RS, Brzyski RG. Effect of chromium supplementation on insulin resistance and ovarian and menstrual cyclicity in women with polycystic ovary syndrome. Fertil steril. 2005;84(6):1755-1757.

27. Wang JG, Anderson RA, Graham GM, 3rd, et al. The effect of cinnamon extract on insulin resistance parameters in polycystic ovary syndrome: a pilot study. Fertil steril. 2007;88(1):240-243.

28. Hlebowicz J, Darwiche G, Bjorgell O, Almer L-O. Effect of cinnamon on postprandial blood glucose, gastric emptying, and satiety in healthy subjects. Amer J Clini Nutr. 2007;85(6):1552-1556.
29. Akilen R, Tsiami A, Devendra D, Robinson N. Cinnamon in glycaemic control: Systematic review and meta analysis. Clin nutr. 2012;31(5):609-615.
30. Khan A, Safdar M, Ali Khan MM, Khattak KN, Anderson RA. Cinnamon improves glucose and lipids of people with type 2 diabetes. Diabetes Care. 2003;26(12):3215-3218.
31. Dugoua JJ, Seely D, Perri D, et al. From type 2 diabetes to antioxidant activity: a systematic review of the safety and efficacy of common and cassia cinnamon bark. Canadian J Physiol Pharmacol. 2007;85(9):837-847.
32. Third Report of the National Cholesterol Education Program (NCEP) Expert Panel on Detection, Evaluation, and Treatment of High Blood Cholesterol in Adults (Adult Treatment Panel III) final report. Circulation. 2002;106(25):3143-3421.
33. Fenugreek. Natural Medicines Comprehensive Database. Accessed January 3, 2013.
34. Baquer NZ, Kumar P, Taha A, Kale RK, Cowsik SM, McLean P. Metabolic and molecular action of Trigonella foenum-graecum (fenugreek) and trace metals in experimental diabetic tissues. J Biosciences. 2011;36(2):383-396.
35. Kannappan S, Anuradha CV. Insulin sensitizing actions of fenugreek seed polyphenols, quercetin & metformin in a rat model. Indian J Med Res. 2009;129(4):401-408.
36. Roberts KT. The potential of fenugreek (Trigonella foenum-graecum) as a functional food and nutraceutical and its effects on glycemia and lipidemia. J Med Food. 2011;14(12):1485-1489.
37. Gupta A, Gupta R, Lal B. Effect of Trigonella foenum-graecum (fenugreek) seeds on glycaemic control and insulin resistance in type 2 diabetes mellitus: a double blind placebo controlled study. J Assoc Physicians India. 2001;49:1057-1061.
38. Zeng T, Guo FF, Zhang CL, Song FY, Zhao XL, Xie KQ. A meta-analysis of randomized, double-blind, placebo-controlled trials for the effects of garlic on serum lipid profiles. J Sci Food Ag. 2012;92(9):1892-1902.
39. Garlic. Natural Medicines Comprehensive Database. Accessed January 12, 2013.
40. Shiyovich A, Sztarkier I, Nesher L. Toxic hepatitis induced by Gymnema sylvestre, a natural remedy for type 2 diabetes mellitus. Amer J Medi Sci. 2010;340(6):514-517.
41. Persaud SJ, Al-Majed H, Raman A, Jones PM. Gymnema sylvestre stimulates

insulin release in vitro by increased membrane permeability. J Endocrinol. 1999;163(2):207-212.

42. Baskaran K, Kizar Ahamath B, Radha Shanmugasundaram K, Shanmugasundaram ER. Antidiabetic effect of a leaf extract from Gymnema sylvestre in non-insulin-dependent diabetes mellitus patients. Journal Ethnopharmacol. 1990;30(3):295-300.

43. Ulbricht C, Abrams TR, Basch E, et al. An evidence-based systematic review of gymnema (Gymnema sylvestre R. Br.) by the Natural Standard Research Collaboration. J Diet Supp. 2011;8(3):311-330.

44. Dona G, Sabbadin C, Fiore C, et al. Inositol administration reduces oxidative stress in erythrocytes of patients with polycystic ovary syndrome. Europ J Endocrinol. 2012;166(4):703-710.

45. Costantino D, Minozzi G, Minozzi E, Guaraldi C. Metabolic and hormonal effects of myo-inositol in women with polycystic ovary syndrome: a double-blind trial. Europ review med pharmacol sci. 2009;13(2):105-110.

46. Unfer V, Carlomagno G, Rizzo P, Raffone E, Roseff S. Myo-inositol rather than D-chiro-inositol is able to improve oocyte quality in intracytoplasmic sperm injection cycles. A prospective, controlled, randomized trial. Europ review med pharmacol sci. 2011;15(4):452-457.

47. Le Donne M, Alibrandi A, Giarrusso R, Lo Monaco I, Muraca U. [Diet, metformin and inositol in overweight and obese women with polycystic ovary syndrome: effects on body composition]. Minerva ginecologica. 2012;64(1):23-29.

48. Venturella R, Mocciaro R, De Trana E, D'Alessandro P, Morelli M, Zullo F. [Assessment of the modification of the clinical, endocrinal and metabolical profile of patients with PCOS syndrome treated with myo-inositol]. Minerva ginecologica. 2012;64(3):239-243.

49. Genazzani AD, Prati A, Santagni S, et al. Differential insulin response to myo-inositol administration in obese polycystic ovary syndrome patients. Gynecol Endocrinol. 2012;28(12):969-973.

50. Gerli S, Papaleo E, Ferrari A, Di Renzo GC. Randomized, double blind placebo-controlled trial: effects of myo-inositol on ovarian function and metabolic factors in women with PCOS. Europ rev med pharmacol sci. 2007;11(5):347-354.

51. Nestler JE, Jakubowicz DJ, Reamer P, Gunn RD, Allan G. Ovulatory and metabolic effects of D-chiro-inositol in the polycystic ovary syndrome. NEJM. 1999;340(17):1314-1320.

52. Baillargeon JP, Iuorno MJ, Apridonidze T, Nestler JE. Uncoupling between

insulin and release of a D-chiro-inositol-containing inositolphosphoglycan mediator of insulin action in obese women With polycystic ovary syndrome. Metabol synd related disorders. 2010;8(2):127-136.

53. Cheang KI, Baillargeon JP, Essah PA, et al. Insulin-stimulated release of D-chiro-inositol-containing inositolphosphoglycan mediator correlates with insulin sensitivity in women with polycystic ovary syndrome. Metabolism. 2008;57(10):1390-1397.

54. Coady MJ, Wallendorff B, Gagnon DG, Lapointe JY. Identification of a novel Na+/myo-inositol cotransporter. Journal bio chem. 2002;277(38):35219-35224.

55. Kennington AS, Hill CR, Craig J, et al. Low urinary chiro-inositol excretion in non-insulin-dependent diabetes mellitus. NEJM. 1990;323(6):373-378.

56. Larner J. D-chiro-inositol--its functional role in insulin action and its deficit in insulin resistance. Intern J experimental diabetes research. 2002;3(1):47-60.

57. Baillargeon JP, Iuorno MJ, Jakubowicz DJ, Apridonidze T, He N, Nestler JE. Metformin therapy increases insulin-stimulated release of D-chiro-inositol-containing inositolphosphoglycan mediator in women with polycystic ovary syndrome. J clin endocrinol metab. 2004;89(1):242-249.

58. D'Anna R, Di Benedetto V, Rizzo P, et al. Myo-inositol may prevent gestational diabetes in PCOS women. Gynecol Endocrinol. 2012;28(6):440-442.

59. Nordio M, Proietti E. The combined therapy with myo-inositol and D-chiro-inositol reduces the risk of metabolic disease in PCOS overweight patients compared to myo-inositol supplementation alone. Europ rev med pharmacol sci. 2012;16(5):575-581.

60. Papaleo E, Unfer V, Baillargeon JP, et al. Myo-inositol in patients with polycystic ovary syndrome: a novel method for ovulation induction. Gynecol Endocrinol. 2007;23(12):700-703.

61. Raffone E, Rizzo P, Benedetto V. Insulin sensitiser agents alone and in co-treatment with r-FSH for ovulation induction in PCOS women. Gynecol Endocrinol. 2010;26(4):275-280.

62. Unfer V, Carlomagno G, Dante G, Facchinetti F. Effects of myo-inositol in women with PCOS: a systematic review of randomized controlled trials. Gynecol Endocrinol. 2012;28(7):509-515.

63. Carlomagno G, Unfer V. Inositol safety: clinical evidences. Euro rev med pharmacol sci. 2011;15(8):931-936.

64. Lee MS, Shin BC, Yang EJ, Lim HJ, Ernst E. Maca (Lepidium meyenii) for treatment of menopausal symptoms: A systematic review. Maturitas. 2011;70(3):227-233.

65. Piacente S, Carbone V, Plaza A, Zampelli A, Pizza C. Investigation of the tuber constituents of maca (Lepidium meyenii Walp.). J ag food chem. 2002;50(20):5621-5625.

66. Feldeisen SE, Tucker KL. Nutritional strategies in the prevention and treatment of metabolic syndrome. Appl Physiol Nutr Metab. 2007;32(1):46-60.

67. Jee SH, Miller ER, 3rd, Guallar E, Singh VK, Appel LJ, Klag MJ. The effect of magnesium supplementation on blood pressure: a meta-analysis of randomized clinical trials. Amer J Hypertension. 2002;15(8):691-696.

68. He K, Liu K, Daviglus ML, et al. Magnesium intake and incidence of metabolic syndrome among young adults. Circulation. 2006;113(13):1675-1682.

69. Kobrin SM, Goldfarb S. Magnesium deficiency. Seminars in nephrology. 1990;10(6):525-535.

70. Guerrero-Romero F, Rodriguez-Moran M. Magnesium improves the beta-cell function to compensate variation of insulin sensitivity: double-blind, randomized clinical trial. Eur J Clin Invest. 2011;41(4):405-410.

71. Mooren FC, Kruger K, Volker K, Golf SW, Wadepuhl M, Kraus A. Oral magnesium supplementation reduces insulin resistance in non-diabetic subjects - a double-blind, placebo-controlled, randomized trial. Diabetes, obesity & metabolism. 2011;13(3):281-284.

72. Song Y, Manson JE, Buring JE, Liu S. Dietary magnesium intake in relation to plasma insulin levels and risk of type 2 diabetes in women. Diabetes Care. 2004;27(1):59-65.

73. Sharifi F, Mazloomi S, Hajihosseini R, Mazloomzadeh S. Serum magnesium concentrations in polycystic ovary syndrome and its association with insulin resistance. 2 Gynecol Endocrinol. 012;28(1):7-11.

74. Kauffman RP, Tullar PE, Nipp RD, Castracane VD. Serum magnesium concentrations and metabolic variables in polycystic ovary syndrome. Acta obstetricia et gynecologica Scandinavica. 2011;90(5):452-458.

75. Magnesium. Natural Medicines Comprehensive Database. Accessed January 16, 2013.

76. Loguercio C, Festi D. Silybin and the liver: from basic research to clinical practice. World J Gastroenterol : WJG. 2011;17(18):2288-2301.

77. Suksomboon N, Poolsup N, Boonkaew S, Suthisisang CC. Meta-analysis of the effect of herbal supplement on glycemic control in type 2 diabetes. J Ethnopharmacol. 2011;137(3):1328-1333.

78. Huseini HF, Larijani B, Heshmat R, et al. The efficacy of Silybum marianum (L.) Gaertn. (silymarin) in the treatment of type II diabetes: a randomized, double-blind, placebo-controlled, clinical trial. Phytotherapy research :

PTR. 2006;20(12):1036-1039.

79. Zapantis A, Steinberg JG, Schilit L. Use of herbals as galactagogues. J Pharmacy Practice. 2012;25(2):222-231.

80. Siriwardhana N, Kalupahana NS, Moustaid-Moussa N. Health benefits of n-3 polyunsaturated fatty acids: eicosapentaenoic acid and docosahexaenoic acid. Advances food nutrition research. 2012;65:211-222.

81. Lopez-Huertas E. The effect of EPA and DHA on metabolic syndrome patients: a systematic review of randomised controlled trials. BJN. 2012;107 Suppl 2:S185-194.

82. Phelan N, O'Connor A, Kyaw Tun T, et al. Hormonal and metabolic effects of polyunsaturated fatty acids in young women with polycystic ovary syndrome: results from a cross-sectional analysis and a randomized, placebo-controlled, crossover trial. Amer J Clin Nutr. 2011;93(3):652-662.

83. Bloch MH, Hannestad J. Omega-3 fatty acids for the treatment of depression: systematic review and meta-analysis. Molecular psychiatry. 2012;17(12):1272-1282.

84. Lin PY, Huang SY, Su KP. A meta-analytic review of polyunsaturated fatty acid compositions in patients with depression. Biological psychiatry. 2010;68(2):140-147.

85. Oner G, Muderris, II. Efficacy of omega-3 in the treatment of polycystic ovary syndrome. J Obstet Gynaecol. 2013;33(3):289-291.

86. Mirmiran P, Hosseinpour-Niazi S, Naderi Z, Bahadoran Z, Sadeghi M, Azizi F. Association between interaction and ratio of omega-3 and omega-6 polyunsaturated fatty acid and the metabolic syndrome in adults. Nutrition. 2012;28(9):856-863.

87. Rizos EC, Ntzani EE, Bika E, Kostapanos MS, Elisaf MS. Association between omega-3 fatty acid supplementation and risk of major cardiovascular disease events: a systematic review and meta-analysis. JAMA. 2012;308(10):1024-1033.

88. Mohammadi E, Rafraf M, Farzadi L, Asghari-Jafarabadi M, Sabour S. Effects of omega-3 fatty acids supplementation on serum adiponectin levels and some metabolic risK factors in women with polycystic ovary syndrome. Asia Pacific J Clin Nut. 2012;21(4):511-518.

89. Cussons AJ, Watts GF, Mori TA, Stuckey BG. Omega-3 fatty acid supplementation decreases liver fat content in polycystic ovary syndrome: a randomized controlled trial employing proton magnetic resonance spectroscopy. J clin endocrinol metabol. 2009;94(10):3842-3848.

90. Vargas ML, Almario RU, Buchan W, Kim K, Karakas SE. Metabolic and endocrine effects of long-chain versus essential omega-3 polyunsaturated fatty acids in polycystic ovary syndrome. Metabolism. 2011;60(12):1711-1718.

91. Akinkuolie AO, Ngwa JS, Meigs JB, Djousse L. Omega-3 polyunsaturated fatty acid and insulin sensitivity: a meta-analysis of randomized controlled trials. Clin nutr. 2011;30(6):702-707.

92. Mehendale SS, Kilari Bams AS, Deshmukh CS, Dhorepatil BS, Nimbargi VN, Joshi SR. Oxidative stress-mediated essential polyunsaturated fatty acid alterations in female infertility. Human fertil. 2009;12(1):28-33.

93. McKeegan PJ, Sturmey RG. The role of fatty acids in oocyte and early embryo development. Repro, fertil, develop. 2011;24(1):59-67.

94. Fish Oil. Natural Medicines Comprehensive Database. Accessed January 8, 2013.

95. Prickly Pear Cactus. Natural Medicines Comprehensive Database. Accessed April 4, 2013.

96. Grube B, Chong PW, Lau KZ, Orzechowski HD. A Natural Fiber Complex Reduces Body Weight in the Overweight and Obese: A Double-Blind, Randomized, Placebo-Controlled Study. Obesity. 2012.

97. Shelton RC. St John's wort (Hypericum perforatum) in major depression. J clin psychiatry. 2009;70 Suppl 5:23-27.

98. Linde K, Berner MM, Kriston L. St John's wort for major depression. Cochrane Database Syst Rev. 2008(4):CD000448.

99. St. John's Wort. Natural Medicines Comprehensive Database. Accessed January 8, 2013.

100. Vassiliadi DA, Barber TM, Hughes BA, et al. Increased 5 alpha-reductase activity and adrenocortical drive in women with polycystic ovary syndrome. J clin endocrinol metab. 2009;94(9):3558-3566.

101. Prager N, Bickett K, French N, Marcovici G. A randomized, double-blind, placebo-controlled trial to determine the effectiveness of botanically derived inhibitors of 5-alpha-reductase in the treatment of androgenetic alopecia. J alt compl med. 2002;8(2):143-152.

102. Saw Palmetto Natural Medicines Comprehensive Database. Accessed January 2, 2013.

103. Holick MF. Vitamin D: importance in the prevention of cancers, type 1 diabetes, heart disease, and osteoporosis. Amer J clin nutr. 2004;79(3):362-371.

104. Lips P. Vitamin D physiology. Progress in biophysics molecular biology. 2006;92(1):4-8.

105. Afzal S, Bojesen SE, Nordestgaard BG. Low 25-Hydroxyvitamin D and Risk of Type 2 Diabetes: A Prospective Cohort Study and Meta-analysis. Clin chem. 2012.

106. Wehr E, Pilz S, Schweighofer N, et al. Association of hypovitaminosis

D with metabolic disturbances in polycystic ovary syndrome. Europ J Endocrinology. 2009;161(4):575-582.

107. Thomson RL, Spedding S, Buckley JD. Vitamin D in the aetiology and management of polycystic ovary syndrome. Clin endocrinol. 2012;77(3):343-350.

108. Firouzabadi R, Aflatoonian A, Modarresi S, Sekhavat L, MohammadTaheri S. Therapeutic effects of calcium & vitamin D supplementation in women with PCOS. Comp ther clin practice. 2012;18(2):85-88.

109. Ardabili HR, Gargari BP, Farzadi L. Vitamin D supplementation has no effect on insulin resistance assessment in women with polycystic ovary syndrome and vitamin D deficiency. Nutr research (New York, N.Y.). 2012;32(3):195-201.

110. Thys-Jacobs S, Donovan D, Papadopoulos A, Sarrel P, Bilezikian JP. Vitamin D and calcium dysregulation in the polycystic ovarian syndrome. Steroids. 1999;64(6):430-435.

111. Lerchbaum E, Obermayer-Pietsch B. Vitamin D and fertility: a systematic review. European J Endocrinol. 2012;166(5):765-778.

112. Ott J, Wattar L, Kurz C, et al. Parameters for calcium metabolism in women with polycystic ovary syndrome who undergo clomiphene citrate stimulation: a prospective cohort study. European J Endocrinol. 2012;166(5):897-902.

113. Grundmann M, von Versen-Hoynck F. Vitamin D - roles in women's reproductive health? Repro bio endocrinol. 2011;9:146.

114. Vitamin D. Natural Medicines Comprehensive Database. Accessed January 16, 2013.

115. Holick MF, Binkley NC, Bischoff-Ferrari HA, et al. Evaluation, treatment, and prevention of vitamin D deficiency: an Endocrine Society clinical practice guideline. J clin endocrinol metab. 2011;96(7):1911-1930.

116. Pacholok S. Could it be B12? Washington, D.C.: Linden Publishing; 2005.

117. Ebbeling CB, Leidig MM, Sinclair KB, Seger-Shippee LG, Feldman HA, Ludwig DS. Effects of an ad libitum low-glycemic load diet on cardiovascular disease risk factors in obese young adults. Am J Clin Nutr. 2005;81(5):976-982.

118. Setola E, Monti LD, Galluccio E, et al. Insulin resistance and endothelial function are improved after folate and vitamin B12 therapy in patients with metabolic syndrome: relationship between homocysteine levels and hyperinsulinemia. European J Endocrinol. 2004;151(4):483-489.

119. Kilicdag EB, Bagis T, Tarim E, et al. Administration of B-group vitamins reduces circulating homocysteine in polycystic ovarian syndrome patients treated with metformin: a randomized trial. Human reprod. 2005;20(6):1521-1528.

120. Mahajan R, Gupta K. Revisiting Metformin: Annual Vitamin B12 Supplementation may become Mandatory with Long-Term Metformin Use. JYP. 2010;2(4):428-429.

121. Tyrer LB. Nutrition and the pill. J Reprod Med. 1984;29(7 Suppl):547-550.

122. Stener-Victorin E, Jedel E, Manneras L. Acupuncture in polycystic ovary syndrome: current experimental and clinical evidence. J neuroendocrinol. 2008;20(3):290-298.

123. Lai MH, Ma HX, Yao H, et al. Effect of abdominal acupuncture therapy on the endocrine and metabolism in obesity-type polycystic ovarian syndrome patients. Acupuncture Res. 2010;35(4):298-302.

124. Lim CE, Wong WS. Current evidence of acupuncture on polycystic ovarian syndrome. Gynecol Endocrinol. 2010;26(6):473-478.

125. Qu F, Zhou J, Ren RX. Effects of acupuncture on the outcomes of in vitro fertilization: a systematic review and meta-analysis. J Alt Compl Med. 2012;18(5):429-439.

Chapter 4

PCOS IN ADOLESCENCE

Sara was 17 years old and had experienced difficulty managing her weight since entering puberty at an early age. She seemed to crave carbohydrates "all the time," even after eating dinner, and complained that her weight had been increasing at a rate of 1 to 2 lbs per month over the past year. Sara had seen a dermatologist for acne on her chin; previously, she had no acne problem. She also had visited her primary care physician for dizziness, feeling shaky, and irregular menses. He started Sara on OCPs to regulate her periods and diagnosed her with hypoglycemia, encouraging her to follow a South Beach-type diet to control her blood sugar and help her lose weight. Nine years later, at age 26, Sara saw an endocrinologist because she could not lose weight, despite her efforts, and because she was experiencing severe hypoglycemia and had elevated serum triglycerides. Sara was diagnosed with PCOS.

THE IMPORTANCE OF EARLY RECOGNITION AND TREATMENT OF ADOLESCENTS WITH PCOS

Adolescence is the most vulnerable and influential stage of PCOS. Signs and symptoms of PCOS usually appear at the onset of puberty when there is a normal increase in insulin levels as part of human development. PCOS is linked to the development of chronic diseases later in life, such as metabolic syndrome, T2DM, heart disease, and endometrial cancer, so early recognition and treatment are critical to prevent these conditions. Since most adult women with PCOS are not diagnosed until after seeking help with infertility, early detection in adolescence could prevent financial and emotional hardships in adulthood.

Gambineri et al showed that middle-aged women with PCOS have a 6.8 times greater chance of developing T2DM than do women without PCOS, and the progression starts early.[1] Adolescents with PCOS who are obese have one-half the peripheral tissue insulin sensitivity than that of adolescents without PCOS who are obese.[2]

Approximately 70% to 74% of adolescents with PCOS are obese.[3] Both obese and nonobese adolescent girls with PCOS have an increased risk of metabolic syndrome compared with girls in the general population.[4-6] Metabolic syndrome is independently associated with sleep-disordered breathing and excessive daytime sleepiness, both of which are highly prevalent in adolescent girls with PCOS.[7]

Additionally, having PCOS may increase the risk of complications during pregnancy, such as GDM, preeclampsia, premature labor, miscarriage, or stillbirth.[8] Early intervention is imperative to prevent these and other conditions by establishing a lifetime pattern of physical activity and healthful eating.[9]

Just as important, many of the signs and symptoms of PCOS can be detrimental to a young woman's quality of life.[10] The most notable of these are weight gain, excessive hair growth on the face and body, "dirty-looking" patches on the skin (acanthosis nigricans), and acne. Such clinical features can significantly impact an adolescent girl's emotional health at a time when self-image is developing and social acceptance is so valued.

Depression and mood disorders are common among adolescent girls with PCOS,[9,11] either because of hormonal imbalances or struggles with body image. Moreover, attempts at weight loss can lead to distorted eating practices or eating disorders; one-third of PCOS women have abnormal eating patterns, and 6% are bulimic.[12]

Some young women with PCOS may feel that having high levels of testosterone and excess weight around their midsection makes them less feminine and more masculine. They may try to "prove" their femininity by being sexually promiscuous, often engaging in unprotected sex to become pregnant, the ultimate sign of femininity.[9,10,13]

Ultimately, the emotional and physical effects of PCOS can extend from adolescence into adulthood.

Because of the vast array of symptoms, PCOS can be difficult to diagnose in adolescence. Dietitians may help assemble the pieces of the puzzle by recognizing the symptoms and encouraging further diagnostic testing. This chapter discusses the challenges of diagnosing PCOS in adolescence as well as treatment strategies.

DIAGNOSING PCOS IN ADOLESCENTS

Though it is increasing known that PCOS exists in adolescents, a knowledge gap remains when it comes to making an accurate diagnosis. Unfortunately, diagnostic criteria for PCOS (see Chapter 1) were developed for the adult woman with PCOS and may not be entirely appropriate for diagnosing PCOS in adolescents. Symptoms of anovulation and hyperandrogenism may vary and appear at different ages among adolescents, if they appear at all. As a result, some researchers have suggested that the diagnostic criteria for PCOS should be different for adolescents.[14]

Table 4.1 shows the typical metabolic and reproductive features in adolescents with hyperandrogenism.

Table 4.1: Hormonal and Metabolic Features in Adolescents with Hyperandrogenism

Free testosterone	↑
Androstenedione	↑ ↔
Dehydroepiandrosterone sulfate (DHEAS)	↑ ↔
Lutenizing hormone (LH)	↑ ↔
Follicle-stiumulating hormone (FSH)	↔
LH/FSH	↑ ↔
Insulin	↑
Insulin-like growth factor binding protein	↓
Sex hormone-binding protein globulin (SHBG)	↓

Reprinted from Warren-Ulanch J, Arslanian S. Treatment of PCOS in adolescence. Best Practice and Research Clinical Endocrinology and Metabolism. 2006;20(2):311-330. Reproduced with permission by Best Practice and Research Clinical Endocrinology and Metabolism. Copyright © 2007.

Insulin Resistance

Insulin resistance is not part of the diagnostic criteria for PCOS but is a classic feature of the syndrome. Acanthosis nigricans is a clinical sign of elevated insulin levels.[9] Dry and rough skin on the elbows, skin tags (also seen with obesity), and rings or lines in the skin around the neck may be seen as well. In fair-skinned women, some of these signs may be difficult to spot.

There is a correlation between an increase in BMI and the severity of insulin resistance in PCOS.[6] Weight found around the midsection with an excess waist-to-hip ratio (greater than 0.85) is attributed to insulin resistance.[13] Accumulation of weight around the abdominal area can be upsetting and frustrating to young women with PCOS, as it may be difficult to lose and sets them apart from their peers.

According to Dr. Katherine Sherif, director of Drexel University's Center for Women's Health and The PCOS Program, insulin acts as an appetite stimulant. "When cells are starved of glucose, as in the case of insulin resistance, they only want more energy, thus stimulating appetite to meet those needs."[15] Adolescent patients (and some adults) seen in my practice have referred to the excess weight as a "spare tire" or "inner tube" around their waist. One teen even named her extra weight, referring to it as "Maurice."

Flannery et al showed an 18.2% prevalence of abnormal glucose metabolism in adolescents with PCOS.[16] Approximately 15.2% of adolescents presented with IGT, independent of BMI.[16] Since insulin resistance is an important risk factor for metabolic syndrome and T2DM, early detection is critical.[6] Screening with a two-hour OGTT is recommended for all adolescents with PCOS, regardless of BMI.[16,17]

Anovulatory Symptoms

Anovulatory symptoms vary and may be classified as amenorrhea (no periods), oligomenorrhea (eight or fewer cycles per year or cycles longer than 40 days), very light flow, dysfunctional uterine bleeding, or heavy periods that can result in anemia.[13,18]

Although menstrual disturbances are perhaps the hallmark feature physicians look for when diagnosing PCOS, it is common for a young woman to experience some form of menstrual disturbances as a natural part of puberty. In fact, by the third year after menarche, 59% of cycles will remain anovulatory in normal females.[19] Therefore, the diagnostic criteria of anovulation or oligoamenorrhea may not always be appropriate in diagnosing adolescents with PCOS.

Unfortunately, many teenagers with oligomenorrhea do not seek help from their physician and, all too often, those who do may be prescribed OCPs to regulate menstrual function instead of being recommended for further endocrine evaluation.[9]

Hyperandrogenism

Hyperandrogenism is classified by acne, hirsutism, and male-pattern baldness or hair thinning.[18] However, just like the other symptoms of PCOS, signs of excess androgen may not appear in all adolescents or may appear at different stages of development with different degrees of severity.[13]

According to Roe and Dokras, hirsutism is a better indicator of hyperandrogenism in teens, as 60% of adolescents with PCOS experience signs of it.[13,14] Since hair growth is less prominent for some girls than adult women, increased serum androgens are the most reliable indicator of androgen excess in the pediatric or adolescent population.[14]

Hyperandrogenism has been proposed to influence intra-abdominal fat because androgen receptors have been located on adipocytes, contributing to the weight-loss difficulties in women with PCOS.[20] In addition, hyperandrogenism has been suggested as an independent risk factor for metabolic syndrome in PCOS,[4] supporting the need for early detection and intervention during adolescence.

Early Puberty and Low Birth Weight

Premature pubarche, or the presence of pubic hair before the age of 8, and a history of low birth weight are risk factors for PCOS.[21] Researchers have found an increased frequency of menstrual dysfunction and hyperandrogenism among girls with premature pubarche who were born at a low birth weight.[22] Premature pubarche is also a risk factor for hyperinsulinemia and dyslipidemia in adolescence.[23]

Sex hormone-binding globulin (SHBG) appears to be lower in girls with premature pubarche.[22] African American and Caribbean Hispanic girls are more prone to developing premature pubarche and PCOS because of earlier and higher levels of androgens.[23] Therefore, these populations should be monitored closely throughout adolescence and early adulthood for insulin resistance and hyperandrogenism.[23]

Polycystic Ovaries

The diagnosis of polycystic ovaries presents unique challenges to diagnosing PCOS in adolescents. Ovarian appearance and volume may change during adolescence. According to Salmi et al, not all women with polycystic ovaries have PCOS, and not all women with PCOS have polycystic ovaries.[9] It is estimated that up to 25% of women without PCOS have cysts around their ovaries.[9] Therefore, despite the syndrome's name, the presence of cysts alone is not sufficient for diagnosis.

It is important to keep in mind that the cysts do not cause PCOS but rather result from hormonal imbalances affecting the ovary; they are not usually painful or dangerous.[18] Ovarian cysts may be part of other conditions, such as congenital adrenal hyperplasia, hypothalamic amenorrhea, or hyperprolactinemia, or just a normal part of puberty.[18,23] Some health care practitioners, along with patients and their families, argue that using a transvaginal approach to detect ovarian cysts in girls is cruel and unnecessary. Transabdominal ultrasound is the preferred method to assess ovarian appearance in girls but is limited in adolescents who are overweight or obese.[14]

Family History
Family history is a risk factor for PCOS in adolescence. First-degree relatives of women with PCOS have higher levels of androgens. In one study, 35% of mothers and 40% of sisters of affected women also had PCOS.[24] Large-for-gestational-age (LGA) girls born to mothers who are overweight or have central obesity and irregular menses are also at risk of developing PCOS.[25]

If PCOS does run in a family, especially if a mother or sister has it, early testing is warranted. Alternatively, if a teen is diagnosed with PCOS, it is also important to screen any of her sisters for it, keeping in mind that symptoms of PCOS vary and appear at different stages of adolescence.

THE DIETITIAN AS DETECTIVE

As dietitians, we have a unique advantage in the ability to recognize PCOS among our adolescent patients because we see patients longer and more frequently. The relationship established with our patients can give us a better sense of their dietary intake, activity levels, cravings, and hunger patterns as well as their feelings toward food and weight. We also have the ability to track patients' symptoms on a more regular basis than other health professionals might. Most commonly, an adolescent, her parents, or her physician will seek advice from a dietitian for help in managing her weight without knowing she has PCOS.

The initial nutrition assessment is an optimal time to quickly screen any female adolescent patient, regardless of her weight status, for possible signs of PCOS. I have found the best time to do this is while inquiring about any medical concerns. I will routinely ask some probing questions pertaining to oligomenorrhea and hirsutism, such as "Tell me what your periods are like. Are they heavy? Irregular? Absent?" and "Can you tell me about any excessive body hair that you may have?"

Depending on the answers to such questions and if the patient does have some irregularity to her periods (especially if they are nonexistent) or has excess weight around her midsection with difficulties losing weight, I will usually probe further, asking the patient if she has ever heard of PCOS or if someone in the family has it. Additionally, I will ask other screening questions, such as "Tell me about any foods that you typically crave" or "Do you ever experience low blood sugar?" More questions can be found in the appendix. Additionally, Table 4.2 lists common indicators of PCOS among adolescents.

Table 4.2: Common Indicators of PCOS Among Adolescents

• Irregular, absent, or heavy menses	• Excess facial hair or hair on other body areas
• Excessive abdominal weight	• Hair loss from head
• Significant weight gain without changes to diet or exercise	• Difficulties losing weight despite efforts
• Skin tags	• Intense carbohydrate cravings
• Acne	• Dark or "dirty-looking" patches on the skin

Sometimes simply asking a patient whether she was ever told that she had abnormal lab results can uncover possible signs of PCOS. I once saw a 15-year-old girl whom I suspected had PCOS because of her struggles with weight, acne, and irregular periods. When I asked her about abnormal lab results, she revealed she had once been told, prior to receiving OCPs to regulate her periods, that she had high testosterone levels, but she had never been diagnosed with PCOS.

Unfortunately, most adult women with PCOS usually have a story to tell about how they finally got diagnosed after seeing numerous doctors throughout their lives, all of whom overlooked their condition. If PCOS is suspected, it is imperative that the dietitian refer the patient to a suitable physician knowledgeable about PCOS for diagnosis and treatment and to rule out any other possible medical conditions. The physician may be a reproductive endocrinologist, endocrinologist, gynecologist, or pediatrician. Patients should always trust their instincts and get a second or third opinion if dissatisfied with their medical care.

TREATMENT OF PCOS IN ADOLESCENTS

Lifestyle modification is the first-line treatment for adolescents with PCOS.[26-28] Adult symptoms of PCOS are known to be alleviated by diet, exercise, weight loss, and androgen- or insulin-lowering medications.[29] However, many of these medications have not been proven safe for adolescents and require compliance. Adolescents generally are more concerned about immediate results and less concerned about improving long-term health. Their reasons for seeking medical care are that they want to lose weight and improve their dermatological symptoms.

The main goals of treatment for an adolescent with PCOS are to regulate menstrual function, reduce androgen and insulin levels, improve dermatological symptoms, and stabilize or reduce weight. Treatment also needs to consider the prevention of long-term health complications as well as the risk for distorted eating and mood disorders. For these reasons, a multidisciplinary team approach involving a pediatrician, dermatologist, endocrinologist, nutritionist, psychiatrist, psychologist, or even a family therapist may be required.

Insulin Sensitizers
Although not yet approved by the FDA for its use among women with PCOS, metformin is the medication most commonly prescribed for treating the syndrome in adults. In addition to improving insulin

sensitivity and glucose metabolism, metformin can ameliorate hyperandrogenism, restore menstrual function, and induce ovulation[30] in women who are lean or obese.[31] Teenagers with PCOS may benefit from the use of metformin, as higher success rates for normalizing menses and improving hirsutism have been found in adolescents than in adults.[30,32,33] Additionally, metformin has been shown to lower total cholesterol, LDL cholesterol, and triglyceride levels in adolescents with PCOS.[22,30,32] Hoeger et al found that metformin, in combination with lifestyle modification, improved central adiposity but did not enhance weight loss in adolescents with PCOS.[34]

According to Rackow,[26] metformin should be used in adolescents who are obese and have been unsuccessful with lifestyle modifications and those with IGT or a strong history of CVD. Patients may not wish to discontinue taking metformin, as doing so has been shown to renew the progression of PCOS symptoms within six months.[22] This reality, along with the disadvantage of a large pill size that can make swallowing difficult, may cause adolescents to discontinue taking metformin or take it inconsistently.

Metformin has been shown to prevent the progression of PCOS in girls as young as 8.[22] Ibanez et al studied the effects of early metformin use (ages 8 to 12) or later use (ages 13 to 14) in girls with premature pubarche and low birth weight.[32] They found that at age 15, girls treated early with metformin had less inflammation and central fat. Hirsutism, androgen excess, oligomenorrhea, and PCOS were more prevalent in girls treated later with metformin. Early treatment with metformin may be used to delay or prevent the onset of PCOS in high-risk girls who have a combined history of premature pubarche and low birth weight.[32]

The investigators suggested that the "window of late childhood and early puberty may be critical for the development and prevention of PCOS."[32] Future studies are needed to address the use of metformin in PCOS as well as the safety of longer-term metformin therapy before puberty, including its possible effects on pubertal growth and development. The possibility that PCOS may be prevented by medication is certainly encouraging.

When working with an adolescent who takes metformin, it is important to let her know in advance that the medication should be taken with food, and diarrhea is a possibility during the first several weeks until her body adjusts to the medication. However, this and other side effects usually subside. An extended-release version of metformin is available and may cause fewer GI side effects.

Patients, especially adolescents, need to know that metformin is not a diet pill, and changes to eating patterns and lifestyle need to be maintained for best results.[34] Supplementation with vitamin B12 is necessary, as metformin causes B12 malabsorption.[35,36]

Oral Contraceptives

Oral contraceptive pills (OCPs) may be used among adolescents to regulate menstrual function and hormone levels as well as improve acne and hirsutism.[9,34] OCPs may be used on their own or in conjunction with metformin and other medications. They may be beneficial for increasing bone density, reducing the risk of endometrial and ovarian cancers, and preventing anemia.[37] Side effects, however, include possible weight gain and increases in triglyceride, cholesterol, and CRP levels,[9,34,38] which can worsen metabolic syndrome risk. In addition, studies have suggested that certain OCPs can decrease insulin sensitivity, thus aggravating impaired glucose metabolism in women who have PCOS,[39] but more research is needed.

Hoeger et al found that OCPs significantly decreased total testosterone (44%) and free androgen index (86%) but also increased CRP (39.7%) and cholesterol (14%) during a 24-week study in teens.[34] OCPs in combination with lifestyle modification had the most benefits in regard to menstrual function and androgen excess in adolescents with PCOS who were obese.[34]

If a teen with PCOS does decide to take OCPs, it is important that she have regular blood work done to monitor changes in lipid levels. In addition to monitoring caloric intake, periodic weight checks may be needed to identify possible weight gain. Supplementation with vitamin B12 may be advised as OCPs have been shown to affect B12 levels.[40]

Antiandrogen Therapy

Acne and hirsutism can significantly affect the body image of a teen with PCOS. Androgen-lowering medications such as spironolactone or flutamide may be prescribed to decrease dermatological symptoms of hair loss and unwanted facial hair[9] and should be initiated early to prevent significant hair growth, which can be longer and more difficult to remove.[18] However, none of these medications are approved by the FDA for the treatment of hirsutism, and most clinical trials evaluating the safety and efficacy of these drugs among adolescents are limited. Additionally, spironolactone should not be taken by women who may become pregnant since it has been linked to birth defects.[18]

Young women prescribed these medications should be educated that it may take three months or longer to see improvements.[23] Other forms of hair removal, such as shaving, electrolysis, and laser therapy, may be safer and faster alternatives.

DIETARY AND LIFESTYLE MANAGEMENT FOR PCOS IN ADOLESCENCE

Lifestyle modification is the preferred and most effective method of treatment for PCOS in adolescence.[9,26-28,31] Weight loss has shown improvements in reproductive and endocrine parameters of PCOS in adults and adolescents, including menstrual function, BMI, and insulin sensitivity.[9,28,41,42] Weight loss due to lifestyle intervention (nutrition education, exercise, and behavior therapy) improved menses, androgens, and cardiovascular risk factors in adolescent girls with PCOS who were obese.[27] Geier et al showed that nearly 70% of adolescents with PCOS succeeded in either weight loss or stabilization when they received treatment from a dietitian and psychologist. [42]

Hoeger et al examined the effects of metformin, OCPs, and/or lifestyle modification in adolescents with PCOS who were obese.[34] Adolescents and their parents participated in a lifestyle modification program that involved a series of classes on diet, exercise, and behavior modification skills along with individual appointments. Lifestyle modification alone resulted in a 59% reduction in free androgen index and a 122% increase in SHBG; results were more significant if weight loss was achieved.

It is interesting to note that the researchers had "significant compliance issues" with adolescents in the lifestyle group,[34] suggesting difficulties sustaining lifestyle changes and counseling this population.

Nutrition management for PCOS is discussed in Chapter 2 but focuses on adults; nutrition information for adolescents with PCOS is limited. Ornstein et al compared the effects of a hypocaloric low-fat diet with a very low-carbohydrate diet in adolescents with PCOS.[28] No significant differences were found; both diets improved BMI, waist circumference, and menstrual function. As the authors pointed out, diet management alone, without the use of insulin sensitizers, can improve menses, weight, and waist circumference in adolescents with PCOS.[28]

Glueck et al found that 2,550 mg of metformin combined with a lower-carbohydrate (less than 44% carbohydrate), calorie-controlled diet (1,200 to 1,800 kcal) improved weight, insulin, dyslipidemia, and menstrual cycles in adolescents with PCOS who were either lean or overweight.[43] More research into the optimal diet for adolescents with PCOS is necessary.

Weight loss improves metabolic and reproductive parameters in adult women with PCOS, but not all women with the syndrome need to lose weight. Because of the scant information available in adolescents, diet recommendations can be applied from women with PCOS, regardless of weight. These recommendations include low saturated fat and carbohydrate intake, predominantly from low-GI foods.[41] The emphasis should be on consuming lean protein sources and unsaturated fats, particularly omega-3 fatty acids.

The importance of eating often (every three to five hours) and including protein with meals and snacks to help manage blood sugar levels and prevent hypoglycemia needs to be stressed to the adolescent with PCOS who, like the majority of adolescents, tends to skip meals or wait long periods between eating. Patients may request a note from their dietitian or physician allowing them to have food in school at times other than lunch because of medical necessity. This can be beneficial considering that for some teens, lunch time is at 10 am.

It is common for women with PCOS to crave carbohydrates more than someone without PCOS. Therefore, some adolescents may find that severely limiting carbohydrates may be too difficult to follow and could contribute to binge eating and weight gain in the long run. Specific information on diet strategies for PCOS can be found in Chapter 2 and the appendix. Additionally, sample meal plans using these recommendations can be found in the appendix.

Reading food labels and using food models are effective ways to teach teens and parents about portion sizes and choosing healthier foods. Meal planning and discussing strategies to cope with social events involving food (e.g., lunch, parties, clubs) are helpful. Some adolescent patients may have an all-or-nothing attitude toward healthful eating for PCOS and need to be reassured that it is acceptable and normal to have some high-fat or highly refined foods once in a while.

Keeping food records can be an effective way for patients to monitor changes in their intake and practice mindful eating. I like to encourage my adolescent patients to experiment with their food choices and see what combinations work best for them.

Some adolescents prefer to use nutritional supplements in the hopes of improving their PCOS symptoms without medications. Others may decide to try nutritional supplements as an adjunct to their current medical treatment. Iron supplementation and iron-rich foods may be recommended to young women experiencing heavy menstrual cycles who have iron deficiency or anemia.

However, the use of nutritional supplements in adolescents is not clearly understood, so they should be used with caution and medically supervised. It is important for patients to consult their physicians prior to taking any nutritional supplement. Even then, careful monitoring for potential side effects or drug-nutrient interactions is warranted. More information on supplements can be found in Chapter 3.

Other Factors to Consider

While weight loss has been shown to improve many symptoms of PCOS, dieting in adolescence is associated with weight gain later in life and an increased risk of eating disorders.[44] Emphasis should be placed on improving adolescents' health by encouraging a healthy approach to eating and exercise rather than focusing on weight loss.

When possible, dietitians should refrain from using calories when counseling their teen patients and avoid classifying foods as "good" or "bad." Because of the higher risk of distorted eating and eating disorders among the PCOS population,[45,46] dietitians need to properly screen adolescent clients for abnormal eating behaviors and attitudes toward food and weight. If distorted eating or an eating disorder is suspected, treatment should be aimed at normalizing eating patterns before recommending changes to eating or activity levels. More information on eating disorders in PCOS can be found in Chapter 8.

Dietitians should take an encouraging, empathetic, and supportive approach when counseling teenagers with PCOS. They need to validate that the weight patients gained was due to hormonal imbalances and not their fault. Patients need to know that they are not alone in their struggles with PCOS symptoms. Many adolescent patients are already concerned about infertility at a young age and need to be reassured that it is possible they will experience no problems conceiving a child. Educating them that improvements in eating and activity patterns can help fertility may be helpful in encouraging adolescents to implement lifestyle changes.

Adolescents and their families need to understand in simplified terms the pathophysiology of PCOS and the connection to their symptoms. They may need education on insulin resistance and why it is important to make lifestyle changes now to prevent further complications. Educating patients on how different foods affect insulin levels may be particularly helpful (e.g., eating whole grain cereal vs. refined grain cereal, eating higher fiber cereal or whole fruit instead of fruit juice).

When counseling adolescent patients, dietitians will also have to address issues with parents. It is common for parents, not knowing their child has PCOS, to assume their daughter is heavy because she has been eating too much. This results in clients feeling blamed and ashamed about their weight, especially if repeated attempts at weight loss have failed.

Parents who try to regulate their daughter's food intake by telling her when to stop eating and what foods she can or cannot have only worsen self-esteem and cause more resentment toward the parents. It also results in teens not being able to effectively trust their internal ability to regulate their food intake. Sometimes teens will admit to sneaking or bingeing on "off-limit" foods to spite their parents. Thus food becomes a tactic used to set boundaries and communication with parents. In these situations, referring patients to an individual or family therapist may be needed. In some instances, dietitians will need to set appropriate boundaries with parents to help them maintain a positive relationship with their daughter.

An important treatment goal is for the teen to assume responsibility for her eating. Parents, who generally do the food shopping and cooking, need to be educated on the proper diet modifications for PCOS and separate myths from facts. In making dietary changes, teens may gain support from family members who may also follow recommended eating plans.[47]

Of course, not all teenagers want to accept responsibility for their eating behaviors or are ready to implement behavioral changes. In these instances, motivational interviewing is an effective counseling technique dietitians can use to help clients work through ambivalence about behavior change.[48] In a nonjudgmental and supportive way, dietitians can help patients explore both positive and negative aspects of their behaviors. By using motivational interviewing techniques such as reflective listening, "rolling with resistance," and positive affirmations, dietitians can avoid getting into power struggles with their adolescent patients and guide them toward change through motivation rather than information.[48] Other counseling styles may be used once the adolescent is ready to implement change.[48]

Physical Activity

Physical activity should be encouraged, as it can improve insulin levels and help manage weight. Exercise can also lower stress and anxiety, prevent chronic disease, and improve body image.

According to government guidelines, adolescents should engage in 60 minutes of physical activity daily. In making recommendations for physical activity, the adolescent's struggle with body image and possible resistance to exercise should be kept in mind. For example, some teenagers who are heavy may avoid swimming because they do not want to be seen in public in a bathing suit, while other activities such as running may be too difficult and embarrassing for them to do.

Ideally, activities that promote skills that can be maintained throughout life should be encouraged. This may include activities such as yoga, Pilates, weight training, tai chi, karate, tennis, golf, bowling, or walking. Nidhi et al showed that yoga improved anxiety,[49] hirsutism, and menstrual frequency[50] as well as glucose, lipid, and insulin parameters in adolescents with PCOS.[51]

Some girls find that they move longer and have more fun when listening to music while exercising.

Dietitians can emphasize that activity in everyday life is important. For example, pedometers can be used to increase walking or climbing stairs rather than taking elevators. Compliance is best when teens can gain support from family members who positively model physical activity themselves.

In summary, PCOS is a complicated endocrine disorder that often goes undiagnosed among adolescents. Teens with PCOS experience many symptoms that can have a significant and long-term impact on self-esteem and body image, putting them at a higher risk of developing an eating disorder. They are also at risk of chronic diseases and infertility later in life. Therefore, early recognition and treatment are key.

Current diagnostic criteria for PCOS may not be appropriate for adolescents, as their symptoms vary at different stages of development and may be seen as a normal part of puberty. Dietitians should screen all their female adolescent patients for PCOS and recommend further diagnostic testing in those they suspect have the syndrome. Once diagnosed, dietitians need to educate patients on the proper dietary management for PCOS and support them in implementing life-long changes to improve their health and prevent chronic disease.

CHAPTER SUMMARY

- Adolescence is the most vulnerable and influential stage of PCOS.
- Many of the symptoms of PCOS are normally experienced during adolescence and can easily be overlooked.
- Diagnostic criteria for PCOS are focused on adults and may not be appropriate for the adolescent population.
- Dietitians should screen all female adolescent patients for PCOS.
- Diet and lifestyle changes are the first-line approach for treating PCOS in adolescence.
- Dietitians need to take an empathetic and encouraging approach to counseling adolescent patients.
- The use of metformin has been shown to improve reproductive and metabolic complications of PCOS among adolescents.
- The use of OCPs should be prescribed to young women with PCOS with caution, as they may negatively affect health.

REFERENCES

1.   Gambineri A, Patton L, Altieri P, et al. Polycystic Ovary Syndrome Is a Risk Factor for Type 2 Diabetes: Results From a Long-Term Prospective Study. Diabetes. 2012.
2.   Ogle A. Before Your Pregnancy: a 90-day guide for couples on how to prepare for a healthy conception. New York, NY: Ballantine Books; 2011.
3.   Yildiz BO, Knochenhauer ES, Azziz R. Impact of obesity on the risk for polycystic ovary syndrome. J Clin Endocrinol. Metab. 2008;93(1):162-168.
4.   Coviello AD, Legro RS, Dunaif A. Adolescent girls with polycystic ovary syndrome have an increased risk of the metabolic syndrome associated with increasing androgen levels independent of obesity and insulin resistance. J Clin Endocrinol Metab. 2006;91(2):492-497.
5.   Hart R, Doherty DA, Mori T, et al. Extent of metabolic risk in adolescent girls with features of polycystic ovary syndrome. Fertil Steril. 2011;95(7):2347-2353, 2353 e2341.
6.   Rahmanpour H, Jamal L, Mousavinasab SN, Esmailzadeh A, Azarkhish K. Association between polycystic ovarian syndrome, overweight, and metabolic syndrome in adolescents. J Pediatr Adolesc Gynecol. 2012;25(3):208-212.
7.   Nandalike K, Strauss T, Agarwal C, et al. Screening for sleep-disordered breathing and excessive daytime sleepiness in adolescent girls with polycystic ovarian syndrome. J Pediatr. 2011;159(4):591-596.
8.   Boomsma CM, Eijkemans MJ, Hughes EG, Visser GH, Fauser BC, Macklon NS. A meta-analysis of pregnancy outcomes in women with polycystic ovary syndrome. Hum Reprod Update. 2006;12(6):673-683.
9.   Salmi DJ, Zisser HC, Jovanovic L. Screening for and treatment of polycystic ovary syndrome in teenagers. Exp Biol Med. 2004;229(5):369-377.
10. Jones GL, Hall JM, Lashen HL, Balen AH, Ledger WL. Health-related quality of life among adolescents with polycystic ovary syndrome. J Obstet Gynecol Neonatal Nurs. 2011;40(5):577-588.
11. Himelein MJ, Thatcher SS. Depression and body image among women with polycystic ovary syndrome. J Health Psychol. 2006;11(4):613-625.
12. McCluskey S, Evans C, Lacey JH, Pearce JM, Jacobs H. Polycystic ovary syndrome and bulimia. Fertil Steril. 1991;55(2):287-291.
13. Thatcher S. Now I'm pregnant. Is the pregnancy at greater risk? In Polycystic Ovary Syndrome: The Hidden Epidemic. Indianapolis, IN: Perspectives Press; 2007.

14. Roe AH, Dokras A. The diagnosis of polycystic ovary syndrome in adolescents. Rev Obstet. Gynecol. 2011;4(2):45-51.

15. Crosignani PG, Colombo M, Vegetti W, Somigliana E, Gessati A, Ragni G. Overweight and obese anovulatory patients with polycystic ovaries: parallel improvements in anthropometric indices, ovarian physiology and fertility rate induced by diet. Hum Reprod. 2003;18(9):1928-1932.

16. Flannery CA, Rackow B, Cong X, Duran E, Selen DJ, Burgert TS. Polycystic ovary syndrome in adolescence: impaired glucose tolerance occurs across the spectrum of BMI. Pediatr Diabetes. 2012.

17. Salley KE, Wickham EP, Cheang KI, Essah PA, Karjane NW, Nestler JE. Glucose intolerance in polycystic ovary syndrome--a position statement of the Androgen Excess Society. J Clin Endocrinol Metab. 2007;92(12):4546-4556.

18. Pfeifer SM. Polycystic ovary syndrome in adolescent girls. Semin Pediatr Surg. 2005;14(2):111-117.

19. Apter D, Vihko R. Premenarcheal endocrine changes in relation to age at menarche. Clin Endocrinol. 1985;22(6):753-760.

20. Moran LJ, Ko H, Misso M, et al. Dietary composition in the treatment of polycystic ovary syndrome: a systematic review to inform evidence-based guidelines. J Acad Nutr Diet. 2013;113(4):520-545.

21. Nicandri KF, Hoeger K. Diagnosis and treatment of polycystic ovarian syndrome in adolescents. Curr Opin. Endocrinol. Diabetes Obes. 2012.

22. Ibanez L, Valls C, Marcos MV, Ong K, Dunger DB, De Zegher F. Insulin sensitization for girls with precocious pubarche and with risk for polycystic ovary syndrome: effects of prepubertal initiation and postpubertal discontinuation of metformin treatment. J Clin Endocrinol. Metab. 2004;89(9):4331-4337.

23. Carlson SE, Colombo J, Gajewski BJ, et al. DHA supplementation and pregnancy outcomes. Am J Clin. Nutr. 2013.

24. Kahsar-Miller MD, Nixon C, Boots LR, Go RC, Azziz R. Prevalence of polycystic ovary syndrome (PCOS) in first-degree relatives of patients with PCOS. Fertil Steril. 2001;75(1):53-58.

25. Brown AJ, Setji TL, Sanders LL, et al. Effects of exercise on lipoprotein particles in women with polycystic ovary syndrome. Med Sci Sports Exerc. 2009;41(3):497-504.

26. Marsh KA, Steinbeck KS, Atkinson FS, Petocz P, Brand-Miller JC. Effect of a low glycemic index compared with a conventional healthy diet on polycystic ovary syndrome. Am J Clin Nutr. 2010;92(1):83-92.

27. Lass N, Kleber M, Winkel K, Wunsch R, Reinehr T. Effect of lifestyle intervention on features of polycystic ovarian syndrome, metabolic syndrome,

and intima-media thickness in obese adolescent girls. J Clin Endocrinol Metab. 2011;96(11):3533-3540.

28. Ludwig DS. The glycemic index: physiological mechanisms relating to obesity, diabetes, and cardiovascular disease. JAMA. 2002;287(18):2414-2423.

29. Kolodziejczyk B, Duleba AJ, Spaczynski RZ, Pawelczyk L. Metformin therapy decreases hyperandrogenism and hyperinsulinemia in women with polycystic ovary syndrome. Fertil Steril. 2000;73(6):1149-1154.

30. De Leo V, Musacchio MC, Morgante G, Piomboni P, Petraglia F. Metformin treatment is effective in obese teenage girls with PCOS. Hum Reprod. 2006;21(9):2252-2256.

31. Tolino A, Gambardella V, Caccavale C, et al. Evaluation of ovarian functionality after a dietary treatment in obese women with polycystic ovary syndrome. Eur J Obstet. Gynecol. Reprod. Biol. 2005;119(1):87-93.

32. Ibanez L, Lopez-Bermejo A, Diaz M, Marcos MV, de Zegher F. Early metformin therapy (age 8-12 years) in girls with precocious pubarche to reduce hirsutism, androgen excess, and oligomenorrhea in adolescence. J. Clin Endocrinol Metab. 2011;96(8):E1262-1267.

33. Moran LJ, Noakes M, Clifton PM, et al. Postprandial ghrelin, cholecystokinin, peptide YY, and appetite before and after weight loss in overweight women with and without polycystic ovary syndrome. Am J Clin Nutr. 2007;86(6):1603-1610.

34. Norman RJ, Davies MJ, Lord J, Moran LJ. The role of lifestyle modification in polycystic ovary syndrome. Trends Endocrinol. Metab. 2002;13(6):251-257.

35. McKeown NM, Meigs JB, Liu S, Saltzman E, Wilson PW, Jacques PF. Carbohydrate nutrition, insulin resistance, and the prevalence of the metabolic syndrome in the Framingham Offspring Cohort. Diabetes Care. 2004;27(2):538-546.

36. Chen ST, Maruthur NM, Appel LJ. The effect of dietary patterns on estimated coronary heart disease risk: results from the Dietary Approaches to Stop Hypertension (DASH) trial. Circ. Cardiovasc. Qual. Outcomes. 2010;3(5):484-489.

37. Hirschberg AL, Naessen S, Stridsberg M, Bystrom B, Holtet J. Impaired cholecystokinin secretion and disturbed appetite regulation in women with polycystic ovary syndrome. Gynecol Endocrinol. 2004;19(2):79-87.

38. Moran LJ, Noakes M, Clifton PM, Wittert GA, Williams G, Norman RJ. Short-term meal replacements followed by dietary macronutrient restriction enhance weight loss in polycystic ovary syndrome. Am J Clin Nutr. 2006;84(1):77-87.

39. Cagnacci A, Paoletti AM, Renzi A, et al. Glucose metabolism and insulin resistance in women with polycystic ovary syndrome during therapy with oral contraceptives containing cyproterone acetate or desogestrel. J Clin Endocrinol Metab. 2003;88(8):3621-3625.

40. Tyrer LB. Nutrition and the pill. J. Reprod Med. 1984;29(7 Suppl):547-550.

41. Marsh K, Brand-Miller J. The optimal diet for women with polycystic ovary syndrome? Br. J. Nutr. 2005;94(2):154-165.

42. Geier LM, Bekx MT, Connor EL. Factors Contributing to Initial Weight Loss Among Adolescents with Polycystic Ovary Syndrome. J. Pediatr Adolesc Gynecol. 2012.

43. Ornstein RM, Copperman NM, Jacobson MS. Effect of weight loss on menstrual function in adolescents with polycystic ovary syndrome. J. Pediatric Adolesc Gynecol. 2011;24(3):161-165.

44. Spear BA. Does dieting increase the risk for obesity and eating disorders? J Am Diet Assoc. 2006;106(4):523-525.

45. Himelein MJ, Thatcher SS. Depression and body image among women with polycystic ovary syndrome. J Health Psychol. 2006;11(4):613-625.

46. Jahanfar S, Maleki H, Mosavi AR. Subclinical eating disorder, polycystic ovary syndrome- is there any connection between these two conditions through leptin- a twin study. Med. J. Malaysia. 2005;60(4):441-446.

47. Jakubowski KP, Black JJ, El Nokali NE, et al. Parents' Readiness to Change Affects BMI Reduction Outcomes in Adolescents with Polycystic Ovary Syndrome. J. Obes. 2012;2012:298067.

48. Kedikova SE, Sirakov MM, Boyadzhieva MV. Leptin levels and adipose tissue percentage in adolescents with polycystic ovary syndrome. Gynecol Endocrinol. 2013;29(4):384-387.

49. Thomson RL, Buckley JD, Brinkworth GD. Exercise for the treatment and management of overweight women with polycystic ovary syndrome: a review of the literature. Obes. Rev. 2011;12(5):e202-210.

50. Nidhi R, Padmalatha V, Nagarathna R, Amritanshu R. Effects of a Holistic Yoga Program on Endocrine Parameters in Adolescents with Polycystic Ovarian Syndrome: A Randomized Controlled Trial. J. Altern. Complement. Med. 2012.

51. Palomba S, Giallauria F, Falbo A, et al. Structured exercise training programme versus hypocaloric hyperproteic diet in obese polycystic ovary syndrome patients with anovulatory infertility: a 24-week pilot study. Hum Reprod. 2008;23(3):642-650.

Chapter 5

PREGNANCY, LACTATION, AND THE POSTPARTUM PERIOD

Pregnancy is an exciting time, especially because so many women with PCOS have been trying to conceive for years with or without fertility treatments. In addition, pregnancy is a definite sign of femininity and may be a relief to some women who have felt masculine over the years due to their "male" shape and symptoms of excess hair growth and balding.

Having PCOS and being pregnant, however, poses additional risks for women with the syndrome. Women with PCOS have an increased risk of GDM and preeclampsia, a syndrome involving hypertension and proteinuria in pregnancy.[1-4] Babies born to mothers with PCOS have an increased risk of being born preterm or LGA and often experience complications during delivery.[4] Women who have undergone fertility treatments may be carrying multiple babies and will have unique dietary and medical concerns.

Proper medical management and MNT are imperative to prevent the onset of these complications and to optimize fetal growth and development. This chapter discusses the nutritional and medical concerns women with PCOS may face during pregnancy and lactation. Suggested dietary interventions for these women are provided. Weight management during the postpartum period is also discussed.

PCOS AND PREGNANCY

Adverse Health Risks of Pregnant Women with PCOS
The NIH defines PCOS as a state of hyperandrogenic chronic anovulation, leading some obstetricians to believe that PCOS does

95

not really exist once a woman becomes pregnant (certainly, they must have ovulated to become pregnant).[5] However, women with PCOS have an increased risk of adverse pregnancy outcomes and should be considered a high-risk group.[4]

Although the exact mechanisms have not been identified, it has long been established that women who are overweight or obese have a higher risk of obstetric and neonatal complications, including GDM,[6] congenital malformations,[6] prolonged labor,[7] cesarean sections,[8-10] macrosomia (infant born weighing more than 4,000 g),[11] preg- nancy-induced hypertension, preeclampsia,[1] and miscarriage.[1,12-15] However, large RCTs have shown that women with PCOS do not have an increased risk of miscarriage.[16]

Since obesity increases obstetric and neonatal risk, interventions aimed at reducing prepregnancy weight and weight management during pregnancy are advised.[14] The Academy of Nutrition and Dietetics and the American Society for Nutrition recommend that all women who are overweight or obese receive nutrition counseling prior to conception and during pregnancy to minimize adverse outcomes.[17]

In a population-based cohort study, Roos et al examined the records of 3,787 births in women with PCOS compared with 1,191,336 births in women without PCOS.[4] PCOS was strongly associated with preeclampsia, and the risk of GDM was more than doubled. Infants born to mothers with PCOS were LGA and had an increased risk of meconium aspiration and low Apgar scores (less than 7) five minutes after birth.[4] These risks were not attributed to maternal weight, advanced age, or reproductive technology. Because BMI was adjusted, the authors suggested that PCOS may increase fetal growth independent of weight.

A 2006 meta-analysis of 720 women with PCOS also found a significant risk of GDM, preeclampsia, and preterm births.[18] The mechanism behind the increased risk of adverse pregnancy and perinatal outcomes is unknown.[4] Increased androgens have been associated with preeclampsia.[19] Elevated maternal insulin and glucose levels may contribute to increased GDM risk.[20]

Gestational Diabetes and PCOS

Gestational diabetes is defined as any degree of glucose intolerance with onset or first recognition during pregnancy.[21] GDM exists in approximately 7% of all pregnancies.[22] Because of the higher rate of obesity, GDM rates are also increasing. New stricter diagnostic criteria for GDM have been proposed and as a result, the number of women with GDM is expected to increase to 18%.[20]

GDM is associated with an increased risk of fetal macrosomia, increasing the need for cesarean births, and maternal hypertensive disorders.[20] Maternal age,[23] obesity, and excessive weight gain increases the risk of GDM.[15,24,25] Long-term risks of GDM include maternal development of T2DM and in babies born to mothers with GDM, an increased risk of obesity, glucose intolerance, and diabetes in late adolescence.[20]

Women with PCOS have an increased risk of developing GDM, independent of weight.[4] Insulin levels significantly increase in the second and third trimesters of pregnancy as a normal part of pregnancy,[17] and the majority of women with PCOS already have hyperinsulinemia. Because of this, glucose testing should be initiated as soon as possible after conception to screen for GDM. If the results are normal, testing should be repeated by the standard screening time for all pregnant women, between 24 and 28 weeks gestation.

A 50-g, one-hour oral glucose challenge is typically first used to screen for GDM in the United States. If high, the American College of Obstetricians recommends the diagnosis of GDM be made based on the result of the 100-g, three-hour OGTT that requires that two or more thresholds be met or exceeded to diagnose GDM.[26]

Glycemic control is essential to prevent complications of GDM, and MNT is the first-line treatment.[27] All women with GDM should receive nutritional counseling from a dietitian on an appropriate diet that provides adequate calories and nutrients for the demands of pregnancy and is consistent with established blood glucose goals.[28] Calorie restriction up to 30% may improve glycemic control and slow the rate of weight gain in women with GDM who are obese.[29] Urinary ketone monitoring can indicate whether the patient is consuming sufficient calories or carbohydrates if she is following a restricted diet.[29] Engaging in consistent, moderate-intensity physical activity may improve insulin resistance and aid in weight management in pregnancy.[30]

If glucose levels do not improve with diet and exercise, insulin or other insulin sensitizers may be needed.[31]

Metformin and Pregnancy

The role of metformin in reducing pregnancy complications in women with PCOS is still controversial. Metformin, a category B drug in pregnancy, is not approved to reduce pregnancy complications. Legro suggested that metformin is prescribed too liberally, as if it is a vitamin that physicians have jumped on the bandwagon to prescribe to women with PCOS without evidence of safety and efficacy.[32] While previous retrospective and nonrandomized studies have shown beneficial effects of metformin on pregnancy loss and complications, only a handful of large RCTs are available.

In their RCT, Vanky et al showed that metformin given during the first trimester (average 10-week gestational age) and continued until delivery did not improve rates of preeclampsia or GDM; metformin use resulted in a near-significant reduction in preterm delivery.[33] Women who took metformin did, however, experience a lower rate of weight gain.[33] A follow-up to another RCT also showed that women who took metformin had less gestational weight gain.[34]

A prospective study involving women with PCOS who received metformin before conception and up to 37 weeks gestation showed a significant reduction in GDM.[35] When Vanky et al reevaluated their findings with an epianalysis, women treated with metformin had a reduced rate of miscarriage and preterm delivery.[36] No difference in the prevalence of GDM and preeclampsia were found with the placebo group.

In their large, randomized, double-blind study, Morin-Papunen et al found that metformin, when given three months prior to conception, improved pregnancy and live-birth rates in women with PCOS.[37] In contrast, a 2012 Cochrane Review showed no evidence that metformin improved live-birth rates.[38]

As previously discussed, women with PCOS have a higher risk of developing GDM. Metformin is believed to reduce the incidence of GDM because of its metabolic, endocrine, vascular, and anti-inflammatory effects.[39] While RCTs are limited, numerous studies have demonstrated that metformin can reduce the incidence of GDM in women with PCOS.[39-41]

Begum et al[41] suggested metformin may reduce GDM in women with PCOS by as much as ninefold. A prospective cohort study found a significant reduction in GDM in women with PCOS who were treated with metformin throughout their entire pregnancy compared with those who stopped metformin around conception.[40] The role of metformin in improving reproductive outcomes requires more RCTs to determine definitive guidelines for its use in women with PCOS.

No evidence of adverse neonatal affects or teratogenicity have been associated with metformin use among women with PCOS.[12] While metformin does cross the placenta, it has not been shown to cause fetal harm.[32,42-44] At dosages between 1.5 to 2.55 g/day, metformin has not been shown to affect newborns' birth weight, length, growth, or motor-social development when 126 infants studied during the first 18 months of life were compared with the normal US infant population.[42]

An RCT showed at that at 1 year of age, infants of mothers who took 2 g/day of metformin were heavier than those in the placebo group (10.2 kg vs 9.7 kg).[34] Metformin exposure was not found to influence growth and body composition at the age of 8.[43] Maternal and newborn androgen and estrogen levels were shown to be unaffected by metformin use in pregnancy.[45]

Weight Gain Recommendations for Women with PCOS

There is a significant amount of literature demonstrating the association between increased complications during pregnancy because of obesity, yet little attention has been given to the management of weight gain during pregnancy. The Institute of Medicine (IOM) has updated its pregnancy weight-gain recommendations based on prepregnancy BMI for women who are overweight or obese. As shown in Table 5.1, women who are overweight should try to gain only 15 to 25 lbs during pregnancy and women who are obese should gain only 11 to 20 lbs.[46] The majority of maternal weight gain should be in the second and third trimesters. Weight-gain recommendations for

Table 5.1: Recommendations for Total Weight Gain During Pregnancy Based on Prepregnancy BMI[46]

Prepregnancy BMI	Total Weight Gain (Singleton)	Total Weight Gain(Multiples)
Underweight (less than 18.5)	28-40 lbs	Insufficient evidence
Normal (18.5 to 24.9)	25-35 lbs	37-54 lbs
Overweight (25 to 29.9)	15-25 lbs	31-50 lbs
Obese (30 or higher)	11-20 lbs	25-42 lbs

women carrying multiples are also shown in Table 1.

Some health care professionals have criticized these guidelines, implying that they are too generous and fail to consider the potential adverse effects of excessive gestational weight gain and do not provide specific recommendations for women with extreme obesity (BMI of 40 or higher).[47,48]

The majority of women exceed the IOM maternal weight gain recommendations.[49-52] One study showed that 57% of white, 61% of black, and 51% of Latina women who were pregnant exceeded the IOM recommendations.[53] Excessive gestational weight gain increases the risk of postpartum weight retention and obstetrical complications such as macrosomia[54] and GDM.[55]

Weight loss is not recommended in pregnancy,[17] and interventions to limit gestational weight gain have demonstrated mixed results.

A systematic review showed that dietary advice during pregnancy is effective for decreasing excessive gestational weight gain and long-term postpartum weight retention but showed limited evidence for benefits on infant and maternal health.[56] Campbell et al found that intense and tailored interventions had no statistically significant effect on gestational weight gain.[57] In contrast, Park et al found low gestational weight gain improved infant and maternal pregnancy outcomes in women with GDM who were overweight or obese.[58]

Dietitians play an important role in providing nutrition counseling to women who are overweight or obese to help reduce the risk of excessive gestational weight gain and improve maternal and infant outcomes. It is important for dietitians to work collaboratively with women with PCOS to prevent excessive gestational weight gain, especially if the patient is overweight or obese prior to conception. Many women who become pregnant may be unaware of the adverse effects of excess gestational weight gain for them or their babies. Interventions that include the use of caloric restriction, diet self-monitoring, self-weighing, exercise, behavior therapy, and regular patient-provider contact may promote weight control in pregnancy, but optimal interventions require more research.[52,59,60]

Emotional Concerns in Pregnancy

Many women with PCOS who can conceive may have misconceptions when it comes to a healthy diet during pregnancy. Although evidence does not support it, popular diet guidelines for PCOS (mostly from the Internet) recommend a very low-carbohydrate diet. This may be problematic for some women who follow these recommendations, as they may feel apprehensive about eating carbohydrate-containing foods during pregnancy. Fruits, vegetables, legumes, and grains provide important vitamins, minerals, and fiber and are essential for fetal growth and development.

Pregnancy is not the time to fear carbohydrates. Women may be inclined to avoid carbohydrates because they think they will gain too much weight or they want prevent the onset of GDM. For these reasons, dietitians should screen pregnant women with PCOS for negative attitudes toward food and weight, separate myths from facts, and recommend appropriate amounts of carbohydrates based on each woman's individual needs.

Some women, on the other hand, may find pregnancy to be a license to eat anything they want as they may, for the first time ever, feel less pressure to restrict their intake in a society obsessed with thinness. This can be troublesome if they have significantly restricted their eating prior to conceiving, as it can lead to bingeing during pregnancy, resulting in excessive weight gain.[30]

Additionally, women who already struggle with anxiety and depression may feel these conditions are exacerbated during pregnancy and could turn to food for emotional support. A study published in the *Journal of the Academy of Nutrition and Dietetics* found that pregnant women who reported high stress, anxiety, and fatigue consumed more carbohydrates, fat, and protein and less vitamin C and folate.[61]

Body image issues can also be a concern during pregnancy, as those who struggled with their weight most of their lives may feel that the weight gain will get out of control. They may also have difficulty accepting weight gain and getting larger in general. Proper education of "where the weight goes" during pregnancy (see Table 5.2) can be helpful to reassure clients that weight gain is necessary and healthy if gained in reasonable amounts.

Women with PCOS tend to carry their weight in their midsection, so they may not look pregnant until their third trimester, causing some to struggle with body image issues of failing to look pregnant. One pregnant PCOS patient I worked with admitted to purposely wanting to eat extra food to gain more weight than she already had because she wasn't "showing" yet and wanted the attention she saw other pregnant women receive. This patient was in the middle of her second trimester and had gained a reasonable 7 lbs.

Dietitians and other health professionals need to screen women with PCOS for possible eating and body image issues to ensure proper fetal growth and development. Patients can benefit from working with a dietitian to understand reasonable weight gain goals, body changes, and eating for a healthy pregnancy.

Table 5.2: Distribution of Total Weight Gain During Pregnancy[62]

Mother		Fetus	
Uterus	2 lbs	Baby	7.5-8.5 lbs
Breasts	1 lb	Placenta	1.5 lbs
Blood	4 lbs	Amniotic fluid	2 lbs
Tissue fluids	3 lbs		
Fat stores	7 lbs		

DIETARY INTERVENTIONS TO IMPROVE MATERNAL AND INFANT OUTCOMES IN PCOS

Women with PCOS should maintain good nutritional status during pregnancy through a lifestyle that optimizes maternal and neonatal health. Women with PCOS have an increased risk of GDM and preeclampsia; a nutrition plan that minimizes these risks and controls for excessive gestational weight gain is advised.

A meta-analysis demonstrated that dietary counseling significantly reduced GDM incidence compared with standard care,[60] emphasizing the need for women with PCOS to receive nutrition counseling during pregnancy.

Caloric Requirements
The phrase "eating for two" is a widespread myth. While an adequate dietary intake for pregnant women is critical for optimal fetal growth and development, consuming excessive amounts of calories is not

ideal. For most women, energy needs during pregnancy range between 2,200 and 2,900 kcal/day. Other factors for determining calorie intake must be considered, including prepregnancy BMI, activity level, rate of weight gain, maternal age, and appetite.[29] Calories should not increase during the first trimester, but government guidelines recommend an extra 340 kcal/day in the second trimester and 452 kcal/day in the third trimester.

According to the Academy of Nutrition and Dietetics, however, some normal-weight and overweight women may not need as many extra calories, especially those who are sedentary.[17] Instead, relying on appetite cues may be a better indicator of energy sufficiency. Ultimately, an individualized approach should determine optimal caloric intake for the appropriate rate of weight gain.

Carbohydrates for Pregnancy

Since there is little data regarding the appropriate dietary pattern for women with PCOS during pregnancy, dietary recommendations must be drawn from other studies involving the effects of carbohydrates on insulin and glucose levels in pregnancy.

Pregnant women should eat a minimum of 175 g of carbohydrates daily[63] to meet fetal brain demands, prevent ketosis, and maintain appropriate blood glucose levels.[64] Consuming too few carbohydrates is not advisable, as they provide energy and fiber as well as essential vitamins and minerals; grains, for example, are important sources of folate. Most importantly, maternal glucose is the primary energy source for intrauterine growth.[63]

The quality and quantity of carbohydrates consumed in pregnancy influences gestational weight gain, glucose tolerance, and possibly birth weight. In an RCT by Walsh et al, 800 women who previously delivered an infant weighing more than 4 kg were chosen to follow a low-GI diet without caloric restriction or to have no diet intervention.[51] Women who followed the low-GI diet had significantly less gestational weight gain (12.2 kg vs. 13.7 kg) and had lower rates of glucose intolerance (21% vs. 28%). No difference in birth weight was found.

A meta-analysis showed low-GI diet advice and an exercise program significantly reduced the risk of macrosomia.[60] Moses et al found a significantly higher prevalence of LGA infants from mothers who followed a high-GI diet compared with those who followed a low-GI diet (33% vs. 3%).[63]

While a low-GI diet may not be the only way to reduce risks, it does offer a simple and safe method for women with PCOS to improve maternal glucose and gestational weight gain.[51]

Maternal consumption of added sugar and sugar-sweetened beverages adversely affect maternal and infant outcomes. The authors of a prospective cohort study suggested that increased sugar intake may directly affect infant birth weight by increasing it.[65] Another prospective study of 32,933 women in Norway showed the intake of added sugar was higher in women who developed preeclampsia than healthy women.[66]

The type and amount of fiber a pregnant woman consumes may reduce the risk of GDM. Epidemiologic data involving 13,110 women from the Nurses' Health Study II showed a 26% reduction in GDM risk for every 10 g/day increase in dietary fiber, a 23% reduced risk for each 5 g/day increase in cereal fiber, and a 26% reduced risk for each 5 g/day increase in fruit fiber.[67] The authors suggested that fiber has a beneficial effect on glucose homeostasis by possibly delaying gastric emptying, which slows glucose absorption and lessens the need for more insulin.[67]

Normally, a state of insulin resistance develops in the third trimester of pregnancy, as higher levels of glucose are utilized to meet fetal demands. Women with low cereal fiber intake and a high GL had a 2.15-fold higher risk of GDM, while women who consumed the most cereal fiber and had the lowest GL experienced the lowest risk of GDM.[67]

It is important for dietitians to encourage pregnant women with PCOS to consume plenty of high-fiber and low-GI foods while avoiding refined carbohydrates and foods and beverages high in sugar. Like nutrition management for GDM, distributing carbohydrates evenly throughout the day to control glucose levels is beneficial, which typically involves consuming three meals and two to four snacks daily, including an evening snack.

Dietary Fat for Pregnancy

Glucose tolerance and GDM also may improve by modifying the type of fat consumed during pregnancy. Low PUFA intake and a low ratio of PUFAs to saturated fat independently predicted glucose tolerance in Chinese women with GDM.[68] The authors concluded that increased PUFA intake is associated with a reduced incidence of glucose intolerance during pregnancy.

Bo et al also found that saturated fat independently affects the development of gestational glucose abnormalities.[69] These findings, however, are not supported by those of Radesky et al, who did not show that nutrient or food intake in early pregnancy is linked to GDM risk.[70] More research on the role of dietary fat in pregnancy is needed.

Consuming adequate amounts of essential fatty acids, particularly EPA and DHA during pregnancy is imperative because they play an important role in infant reproductive, brain, immune, and visual function, and may reduce the incidence of pregnancy-induced hypertension.[71]

Currently, during pregnancy, the DRI for linoleic acid (omega-6 fatty acids) is 13 g and 1.4 grams for alpha-linolenic acid (omega-3 fatty acids).[72] Worldwide, there is an increased intake of omega-6 fatty acids and an inadequate intake of omega-3 fatty acids.[73] Additionally, vegetarians may have inadequate omega-3 fat intake, and lower levels of DHA have been reported in infants born to vegetarian mothers.[74]

Good sources of omega-3 fats that are safe for women to eat during pregnancy include freshly ground flaxseeds and unprocessed flaxseed oil, walnuts, butternuts, cold-pressed and unrefined canola and soybean oils, cold-water fish (limited to 12 oz per week), egg yolks, and organ meats. Additionally, many prenatal vitamins now include omega-3 fatty acids, which can help increase intake. Although a good source of omega-3 fats, cod liver oil should be avoided in pregnancy because of its potentially high vitamin A content.[75]

Both omega-6 and omega-3 fatty acid levels decrease significantly during pregnancy, as women have difficulty keeping up with the high demand, especially for DHA, which is important for brain and vision development, and EPA, which promotes immune function.[71,73] The more fetuses a woman carries, the more essential fatty acids she loses.[73] Once stores are compromised, they are slow to recover unless extra supplementation is given.[71]

For these reasons, pregnant women should consume sufficient essential fatty acids to meet their needs and those of their fetus (or fetuses).[71,73,76] Supplementation with 600 mg of DHA per day in the last half of pregnancy resulted in overall greater gestation duration and infant size.[77]

In addition, it may be beneficial for women to continue supplementing their diets with omega-3 fatty acids for the first six months after giving birth.[71] Future research is needed to determine optimal dosage amounts.[71]

Nutritional Supplements and Disease Risk

Calcium supplementation may reduce the risk of gestational hypertension or preeclampsia. Two meta-analyses showed that additional calcium intake during pregnancy is effective for reducing the incidence of preeclampsia, especially in populations where calcium intake is low.[78,79] Calcium supplementation was also shown to reduce the risk of preterm births.[79]

Meta-analyses showed interventions with vitamin C alone or combined with vitamin E did not reduce the incidence of preeclampsia, premature membrane rupture, or other adverse pregnancy outcomes.[80,81] Vitamin D, however, is associated with a reduced risk of preeclampsia in women with poor vitamin D levels.[82]

The Use of Alternative Remedies in Pregnancy

It is popular among women with PCOS to take herbal and botanical products to treat symptoms and possibly increase fertility. Some women may wish to continue taking them during pregnancy, especially if they deem them safe or natural. Those who could conceive while taking alternative treatments may want to continue taking them in the hopes the supplements will help support a healthy pregnancy.

As mentioned in Chapter 3, the safety and effectiveness of the majority of these products have not been studied in pregnant and lactating women, and they should be viewed as drugs. Many of these herbs, such as black cohosh, chasteberry, and fenugreek, can alter hormone levels and stimulate uterine contractions. A list of some common herbs and botanicals contraindicated in pregnancy are listed in Table 5.3.

Exercise in Pregnancy

It is recommended that pregnant women engage in at least 30 minutes of moderate physical activity on most days of the week.[29] Pregnant women with PCOS can reap the benefits of physical exercise, including weight management, increased physical fitness (likely to help with the

Table 5.3: Some Herbal and Botanical Supplements
to Avoid During Pregnancy[83,84]

Agnus castus	Black cohosh	Dong quai
Ginseng	Licorice	Sassafras
Cayenne pepper	Blue cohosh	Echinacea
Feverfew	Motherwort	St. John's wort
Chamomile	Comfrey	Fenugreek
Hawthorne	Red clover	Valerian root
Fennel	Vervain	

demands of labor and recovery), reduced risk of developing GDM and pregnancy-induced hypertension, and psychological well-being.[29] In addition, moderate physical activity during pregnancy has been shown to lower maternal glucose levels in women with GDM.[22] Women who did not exercise prior to pregnancy should consult with their obstetrician before starting an exercise program.

PCOS AND LACTATION

Do Women With PCOS Have More Difficulty Breast-Feeding?

Because of the many hormonal imbalances associated with PCOS, it has been speculated that some women with the syndrome may have difficulty breast-feeding and producing an adequate milk supply for their infants. The hormonal aberrations in PCOS involve insulin, progesterone, and estrogen, all of which are important to breast development and milk secreting ability.[85]

Lactation consultant Lisa Marasco, MA, IBCLC, began studying the connection between PCOS and low milk supply after seeing two PCOS patients within one day who had problems with low milk production. In her thesis, she studied a group of 30 women with lactation failure and found that more than one-half of them were obese, 57% had a history of infertility, and 67% experienced oligo- or amenorrhea.[85]

According to Marasco, some women with PCOS may experience more difficulty producing adequate milk because the breast tissue fails to undergo the normal physiological changes during pregnancy needed to prepare for lactation or not enough breast tissue existed prior to pregnancy.[86] In an RCT, women with PCOS who had no change in breast size during pregnancy were more likely to be obese and have higher blood pressure, triglyceride, and fasting insulin levels.[87]

Additionally, it is known that women with PCOS have low levels of progesterone, which is needed for alveolar growth and development in breast tissue. Insulin also plays a role in milk production, and having hyperinsulinemia may contribute to lactation problems in women with PCOS.[85]

Some lactation consultants recommend that all women with PCOS pump after feedings for at least 10 to 15 minutes on each breast to help establish an adequate milk supply in the first two weeks of initiating nursing. Frequent feedings with full drainage can also help maximize milk production as well as drinking at least sixteen 8-oz glasses of water (16 oz at each nursing session) each day and eating an adequate diet. (One study showed that the volume of milk production decreases when caloric intake drops below 1,500 kcal/day.[88]) For mothers with a low milk supply, extra breast stimulation by frequent nursing or pumping sessions is crucial.

Milk supply problems may be prevented or ameliorated by establishing early intervention strategies during pregnancy. This may include obtaining resources for local breast-feeding support groups and preparing to work with a board-certified lactation consultant soon after giving birth. Good breast-feeding management, including proper latching and positioning, are imperative to successful milk production and proper infant growth and development.

According to Marasco, these tactics will help establish the foundation for a good milk supply, yet they do not address the underlying problems.[86]

Although not scientifically tested, goat's rue, fennel, kale, verbena, chasteberry, and fenugreek are herbal supplements reputed to increase milk supply and possibly stimulate breast growth.[85,89] The use of progesterone supplements and metformin during pregnancy have also been speculated to help support an adequate milk supply in women with PCOS and possibly support breast development during pregnancy but also has not been proven.[85,90]

Marasco claims she has tried metformin with "a number of PCOS moms with low supply and, in some cases, metformin alone increases milk production."[85] But, she adds, "Metformin is not going to help much if the woman does not have enough breast tissue in place to begin with."[86] Medications such as metoclopramide (Reglan) can also be prescribed to boost milk supply.[85,86]

Interestingly, while some women with PCOS experience low milk supply, others report an overabundance of milk production. Obviously, this is an area that requires more attention.

Is Metformin Safe to Use while Breast-Feeding?

Women with PCOS may choose to take metformin during pregnancy and may be inclined to continue taking metformin while they breast-feed to prevent the "rebounding" of PCOS symptoms after birth, control insulin levels, and possibly improve milk supply. However, the use of metformin during lactation is still controversial.

Not surprisingly, limited information exists about whether metformin is safe to take while breast-feeding, as the risks to the infant are still unknown. The few studies that are available have consisted of relatively limited sample sizes. Results showed that metformin does cross into the milk supply but in amounts that appear to be clinically insignificant, with no adverse affects to infants.[89,91-93]

The largest study to date was conducted among 61 nursing infants and 50 formula-fed infants born to mothers with PCOS who took an average of 2.55 g of metformin per day throughout pregnancy and lactation.[94] The infants were followed up to 6 months of age, with results showing that the breast-fed infants of mothers who took metformin had no adverse health risks in regard to growth or motor-social development.[95]

In researching this book, however, the numerous pediatricians, obstetricians, and reproductive endocrinologists I interviewed have offered conflicting advice on whether to take metformin while nursing. Some physicians do not feel comfortable advising women to breast-feed while taking the medication because of the lack of evidence supporting the safety of metformin while breast-feeding. Other physicians said they have been instructing moms to breast-feed while taking metformin, as infants have already been exposed to it in utero and because it does not appear to be teratogenic, cause hypoglycemia, or lead to other adverse health risks.[95-97]

Basically, until more larger long-term studies are conducted, women with PCOS who do plan to breast-feed and take metformin should discuss their options with their physician and carefully make a risk-benefit analysis before beginning breast-feeding. If a woman does decide to take metformin while nursing, frequent monitoring of the infant's health and feeding habits are advisable.[92,93]

POSTPARTUM WEIGHT MANAGEMENT FOR MOTHERS WITH PCOS

Studies suggest that the greater amount of weight a women gains during her pregnancy, the more likely she is to retain the weight postpartum.[98,99] Being at a higher weight between pregnancies may contribute to complications in subsequent pregnancies, lead to weight retention throughout life, and contribute to obesity. There is limited information as to the hormonal effects a woman with PCOS will endure during her postpartum period. One study showed lactation did not improve insulin resistance in women with PCOS.[100]

Lactation may help healthy women lose weight after childbirth because of the increased amount of calories burned (on average, 500 kcal/day for a normal-weight woman in the first six months) because there is a higher demand for glucose by the mammary gland. It is unknown whether this is true in PCOS.

There are many factors that can affect weight-loss efforts in the postpartum period. One main obstacle is lack of sleep. Anyone reading this who has children can relate to the many sleepless nights common during a baby's first few months. Insufficient sleep is related to weight gain and hormonal changes. In fact, sleep deprivation has been associated with decreased leptin and increased ghrelin, both of which may stimulate hunger and appetite, especially for high-carbohydrate and energy-dense foods.[101] This can be problematic for women with PCOS because such foods can negatively affect insulin levels and lead to weight gain.

Additionally, some women may find themselves engaging in binge or emotional eating during sleepless nights when they are up caring for their baby, which can also contribute to weight gain and resistance to postpartum weight loss. Dietitians can help women become more aware of their emotional triggers and identify healthy ways of coping with their emotions other than turning to food for support.

Lack of exercise is another factor contributing to postpartum weight retention. Finding time for physical activity with a newborn can be particularly challenging without proper support. Discussing plans for physical activity after childbirth may help with compliance. Ideas for new mothers include exercising at home with equipment or DVDs, joining exercise classes that involve the baby, finding areas they can walk with the baby in a stroller or carrier, or deciding who may watch their child during exercise, perhaps utilizing childcare services at a gym.

The added responsibility and time demands of caring for a newborn can affect a woman's ability to make wise food choices and purchase and prepare healthier meals. It could also affect a woman's ability to respond to her own needs for food because she can't always eat when she needs to.

According to Debra Krummel, PhD, RD, the first step in providing nutrition counseling to a woman for postpartum weight management is to assess the client's readiness, intention, and barriers to change.[50] This will help the dietitian and the patient decide what steps need to be followed for change to occur.

The use of motivational interviewing as well as regular counseling sessions can be beneficial. Providing patients with a meal plan consisting of appropriate daily calorie goals and education on portion sizes can be beneficial for postpartum weight loss, especially since women may have been accustomed to eating a higher calorie intake during pregnancy.

It is important to have a sufficient food supply at home, including items that can easily be prepared. Patients can be encouraged to accept support from family and friends who want to help with grocery shopping and meal preparation. Stocking the freezer with vegetables and healthy homemade meals prepared during pregnancy, for example, can also be useful.

In summary, though pregnancy is a time of joy, it poses additional health risks for women with PCOS; pregnancy in women with the condition should be considered high risk. Some women may resist eating carbohydrates or consume too many during pregnancy, posing additional risks to both mother and baby.

Dietitians need to educate women on the benefits of a healthy diet and lifestyle to sustain a healthy pregnancy and prevent complications, including providing information about the appropriate amount and pacing of weight gain.

Women with PCOS may have concerns during the postpartum period that could affect lactation, eating habits, and overall weight management. MNT, therefore, plays an integral part in the health of women with PCOS during pregnancy and throughout the postpartum period.

CHAPTER SUMMARY

- Women with PCOS have an increased risk of GDM, preterm births, preeclampsia, and LGA infants.
- Glucose screening should be initiated as soon as possible after conception to screen for GDM.
- Dietitians need to educate women on the benefits of a healthy diet and lifestyle to sustain a healthy pregnancy, including information on the appropriate amount and pacing of weight gain.
- Dietitians should encourage patients with PCOS to consume whole grain and high-fiber foods, including breads, cereals, fruits, legumes, and vegetables.
- Refined carbohydrates, including sweets and sweetened beverages, should be avoided in pregnancy.
- Taking metformin during pregnancy reduces the risk of GDM and prevents excessive gestational weight gain.
- Hormonal imbalances in PCOS may affect nursing moms' ability to establish adequate breast development and milk production.
- Working with a board-certified lactation consultant and using herbal or medical treatments may help increase milk supply.
- A number of obstacles can affect postpartum weight loss, including sleep deprivation, stress, dietary changes, and lack of exercise.

REFERENCES

1. Florakis D, Diamanti-Kandarakis E, Katsikis I, et al. Effect of hypocaloric diet plus sibutramine treatment on hormonal and metabolic features in overweight and obese women with polycystic ovary syndrome: a randomized, 24-week study. Int. J. Obes. 2008;32(4):692-699.

2. Bradley U, Spence M, Courtney CH, et al. Low-fat versus low-carbohydrate weight reduction diets: effects on weight loss, insulin resistance, and cardiovascular risk: a randomized control trial. Diabetes. 2009;58(12):2741-2748.

3. Kogure GS, Piccki FK, Vieira CS, Martins Wde P, dos Reis RM. [Analysis of muscle strength and body composition of women with polycystic ovary syndrome]. Rev. Bras. Ginecol. Obstet. 2012;34(7):316-322.

4. Roos N, Kieler H, Sahlin L, Ekman-Ordeberg G, Falconer H, Stephansson O. Risk of adverse pregnancy outcomes in women with polycystic ovary syndrome: population based cohort study. BMJ. 2011;343:d6309.

5. Thatcher S. Now I'm pregnant. Is the pregnancy at greater risk? In Polycystic Ovary Syndrome: The Hidden Epidemic. Indianapolis, IN: Perspectives Press; 2007.

6. de Punder K, Pruimboom L. The Dietary Intake of Wheat and other Cereal Grains and Their Role in Inflammation. Nutrients. 2013;5(3):771-787.

7. Gambarin-Gelwan M, Kinkhabwala SV, Schiano TD, Bodian C, Yeh HC, Futterweit W. Prevalence of nonalcoholic fatty liver disease in women with polycystic ovary syndrome. Clin. Gastroenterol. Hepatol. 2007;5(4):496-501.

8. Cnattingius S, Bergstrom R, Lipworth L, Kramer MS. Prepregnancy weight and the risk of adverse pregnancy outcomes. The New England journal of medicine. 1998;338(3):147-152.

9. Parker HM, Johnson NA, Burdon CA, Cohn JS, O'Connor HT, George J. Omega-3 supplementation and non-alcoholic fatty liver disease: a systematic review and meta-analysis. J. Hepatol. 2012;56(4):944-951.

10. El-Mesallamy HO, Abd El-Razek RS, El-Refaie TA. Circulating high-sensitivity C-reactive protein and soluble CD40 ligand are inter-related in a cohort of women with polycystic ovary syndrome. Eur. J. Obstet. Gynecol. Reprod. Biol. 2013.

11. Biesiekierski JR, Newnham ED, Irving PM, et al. Gluten causes gastrointestinal symptoms in subjects without celiac disease: a double-blind randomized placebo-controlled trial. Am. J. Gastroenterol. 2011;106(3):508-514; quiz 515.

12. Adebamowo CA, Spiegelman D, Danby FW, Frazier AL, Willett WC, Holmes MD. High school dietary dairy intake and teenage acne. J. Am. Acad. Dermatol. 2005;52(2):207-214.

13. Chavarro J, Willet, W. The Fertility Diet. New York, NY: McGraw Hill; 2007.

14. Cuff DJ, Meneilly GS, Martin A, Ignaszewski A, Tildesley HD, Frohlich JJ. Effective exercise modality to reduce insulin resistance in women with type 2 diabetes. Diabetes Care. 2003;26(11):2977-2982.

15. Dennedy MC, Avalos G, O'Reilly MW, O'Sullivan EP, Dunne FP. The impact of maternal obesity on gestational outcomes. Irish medical journal. 2012;105(5 Suppl):23-25.

16. Legro RS, Barnhart HX, Schlaff WD, et al. Clomiphene, metformin, or both for infertility in the polycystic ovary syndrome. The New England journal of medicine. 2007;356(6):551-566.

17. Siega-Riz AM, King JC. Position of the American Dietetic Association and American Society for Nutrition: obesity, reproduction, and pregnancy outcomes. Journal of the American Dietetic Association. 2009;109(5): 918-927.

18. Boomsma CM, Eijkemans MJ, Hughes EG, Visser GH, Fauser BC, Macklon NS. A meta-analysis of pregnancy outcomes in women with polycystic ovary syndrome. Hum. Reprod. Update. 2006;12(6):673-683.

19. Troisi R, Potischman N, Roberts J, et al. Associations of maternal and umbilical cord hormone concentrations with maternal, gestational and neonatal factors. CCC. 2003;14(4):347-355.

20. Hyperglycemia and Adverse Pregnancy Outcomes. NEJM. 2008;358(19): 1991-2002.

21. Douglas CC, Norris LE, Oster RA, Darnell BE, Azziz R, Gower BA. Difference in dietary intake between women with polycystic ovary syndrome and healthy controls. Fertil. Steril. 2006;86(2):411-417.

22. Gestational Diabetes Mellitus. Diabetes Care. 2003;26(suppl 1):s103-s105.

23. Shrestha A, Chawla CD. The glucose challenge test for screening of gestational diabetes. KUMJ. 2011;9(34):22-25.

24. Baci Y, Ustuner I, Keskin HL, Ersoy R, Avsar AF. Effect of maternal obesity and weight gain on gestational diabetes mellitus. Gynecol endocrinol. 2012.

25. Carreno CA, Clifton RG, Hauth JC, et al. Excessive early gestational weight gain and risk of gestational diabetes mellitus in nulliparous women. Obstet gynecol. 2012;119(6):1227-1233.

26. ACOG Practice Bulletin. Clinical management guidelines for obstetrician-gynecologists. Number 30, September 2001 (replaces Technical Bulletin Number 200, December 1994). Gestational diabetes. Obstet gynecol. 2001;98(3):525-538.

27. Franz MJ, Bantle JP, Beebe CA, et al. Evidence-based nutrition principles

and recommendations for the treatment and prevention of diabetes and related complications. Diabetes Care. 2003;26 Suppl 1:S51-61.

28. Standards of medical care in diabetes--2012. Diabetes Care. 2012;35 Suppl 1:S11-63.

29. Kaiser L, Allen LH. Position of the American Dietetic Association: nutrition and lifestyle for a healthy pregnancy outcome. J Amer Diet Assoc. 2008;108(3):553-561.

30. Mumford SL, Siega-Riz AM, Herring A, Evenson KR. Dietary restraint and gestational weight gain. J Amer Diet Assoc. 2008;108(10):1646-1653.

31. Refuerzo JS. Oral hypoglycemic agents in pregnancy. Obstetrics and gynecology clinics of North America. 2011;38(2):227-234.

32. Legro RS. Metformin during pregnancy in polycystic ovary syndrome: another vitamin bites the dust. J clin endocrinol metabolism. 2010;95(12):5199-5202.

33. Vigorito C, Giallauria F, Palomba S, et al. Beneficial effects of a three-month structured exercise training program on cardiopulmonary functional capacity in young women with polycystic ovary syndrome. J Clin Endocrinol Metab. 2007;92(4):1379-1384.

34. Carlsen SM, Martinussen MP, Vanky E. Metformin's Effect on First-Year Weight Gain: A Follow-up Study. Pediatrics. 2012;130(5):e1222-1226.

35. De Leo V, Musacchio MC, Piomboni P, Di Sabatino A, Morgante G. The administration of metformin during pregnancy reduces polycystic ovary syndrome related gestational complications. Euro J Obstetrics, Gynecology, Reprod Bio. 2011;157(1):63-66.

36. Vanky E, F DEZ, Diaz M, Ibanez L, Carlsen SM. On the potential of metformin to prevent preterm delivery in women with polycystic ovary syndrome - an epi-analysis. Acta obstetricia et gynecologica. 2012.

37. Morin-Papunen L, Rantala AS, Unkila-Kallio L, et al. Metformin improves pregnancy and live-birth rates in women with polycystic ovary syndrome (PCOS): a multicenter, double-blind, placebo-controlled randomized trial. J Clin Endocrinol Metab. 2012;97(5):1492-1500.

38. Tang T, Lord JM, Norman RJ, Yasmin E, Balen AH. Insulin-sensitising drugs (metformin, rosiglitazone, pioglitazone, D-chiro-inositol) for women with polycystic ovary syndrome, oligo amenorrhoea and subfertility. Cochrane Database Syst Rev. 2012;5:CD003053.

39. Kumar P, Khan K. Effects of metformin use in pregnant patients with polycystic ovary syndrome. J Human Reprod Sciences. 2012;5(2):166-169.

40. Khattab S, Mohsen IA, Aboul Foutouh I, et al. Can metformin reduce

the incidence of gestational diabetes mellitus in pregnant women with polycystic ovary syndrome? Prospective cohort study. Gynecol Endocrinol. 2011;27(10):789-793.

41. Begum MR, Khanam NN, Quadir E, et al. Prevention of gestational diabetes mellitus by continuing metformin therapy throughout pregnancy in women with polycystic ovary syndrome. Journal Obstet Gynaecol Res. 2009;35(2):282-286.

42. Glueck CJ, Goldenberg N, Pranikoff J, Loftspring M, Sieve L, Wang P. Height, weight, and motor-social development during the first 18 months of life in 126 infants born to 109 mothers with polycystic ovary syndrome who conceived on and continued metformin through pregnancy. Human reprod. 2004;19(6):1323-1330.

43. Moran LJ, Harrison CL, Hutchison SK, Stepto NK, Strauss BJ, Teede HJ. Exercise decreases anti-mullerian hormone in anovulatory overweight women with polycystic ovary syndrome: a pilot study. Horm. Metab. Res. 2011;43(13):977-979.

44. Rowan JA, Rush EC, Obolonkin V, Battin M, Wouldes T, Hague WM. Metformin in gestational diabetes: the offspring follow-up (MiG TOFU): body composition at 2 years of age. Diabetes Care. 2011;34(10):2279-2284.

45. Carlsen SM, Vanky E. Metformin influence on hormone levels at birth, in PCOS mothers and their newborns. Human reprod. 2010;25(3):786-790.

46. Guidelines CtRIPW, Medicine Io, Council NR. Weight Gain During Pregnancy: Reexamining the Guidelines. The National Academies Press; 2009.

47. Vujkovic M, de Vries JH, Lindemans J, et al. The preconception Mediterranean dietary pattern in couples undergoing in vitro fertilization/ intracytoplasmic sperm injection treatment increases the chance of pregnancy. Fertil. Steril. 2010;94(6):2096-2101.

48. Qin B, Panickar KS, Anderson RA. Cinnamon: potential role in the prevention of insulin resistance, metabolic syndrome, and type 2 diabetes. J Diabetes Sci Technol. 2010;4(3):685-693.

49. Bird ST, Hartzema AG, Brophy JM, Etminan M, Delaney JA. Risk of venous thromboembolism in women with polycystic ovary syndrome: a population-based matched cohort analysis. CMAJ. 2013;185(2):E115-120.

50. Chavarro JE, Rich-Edwards JW, Rosner BA, Willett WC. Diet and lifestyle in the prevention of ovulatory disorder infertility. Obstet. Gynecol. 2007;110(5):1050-1058.

51. Walsh JM, McGowan CA, Mahony R, Foley ME, McAuliffe FM. Low

glycaemic index diet in pregnancy to prevent macrosomia (ROLO study): randomised control trial. BMJ. 2012;345:e5605.

52. Kinnunen TI, Raitanen J, Aittasalo M, Luoto R. Preventing excessive gestational weight gain-a secondary analysis of a cluster-randomised controlled trial. Euro Clinical Nutr. 2012;66(12):1344-1350.

53. Chavarro JE, Rich-Edwards JW, Rosner B, Willett WC. A prospective study of dairy foods intake and anovulatory infertility. Hum. Reprod. 2007;22(5):1340-1347.

54. Galtier-Dereure F, Boegner C, Bringer J. Obesity and pregnancy: complications and cost. Amer J Clin Nutr. 2000;71(5 Suppl):1242S-1248S.

55. Morisset AS, St-Yves A, Veillette J, Weisnagel SJ, Tchernof A, Robitaille J. Prevention of gestational diabetes mellitus: a review of studies on weight management. Diabetes/metabolism research and reviews. 2010;26(1):17-25.

56. Tanentsapf I, Heitmann BL, Adegboye AR. Systematic review of clinical trials on dietary interventions to prevent excessive weight gain during pregnancy among normal weight, overweight and obese women. BMC pregnancy and childbirth. 2011;11:81.

57. Campbell F, Johnson M, Messina J, Guillaume L, Goyder E. Behavioural interventions for weight management in pregnancy: a systematic review of quantitative and qualitative data. BMC public health. 2011;11:491.

58. Park JE, Park S, Daily JW, Kim SH. Low gestational weight gain improves infant and maternal pregnancy outcomes in overweight and obese Korean women with gestational diabetes mellitus. Gynecolog Endocrinol. 2011;27(10):775-781.

59. Phelan S, Jankovitz K, Hagobian T, Abrams B. Reducing excessive gestational weight gain: lessons from the weight control literature and avenues for future research. Women's health. 2011;7(6):641-661.

60. Oostdam N, van Poppel MN, Wouters MG, van Mechelen W. Interventions for preventing gestational diabetes mellitus: a systematic review and meta-analysis. J Women's Health (2002). 2011;20(10):1551-1563.

61. Bruner B, Chad K, Chizen D. Effects of exercise and nutritional counseling in women with polycystic ovary syndrome. Appl Physiol Nutr Metab. 2006;31(4):384-391.

62. Moran LJ, Brinkworth G, Noakes M, Norman RJ. Effects of lifestyle modification in polycystic ovarian syndrome. Reprod Biomed Online. 2006;12(5):569-578.

63. Oner G, Muderris, II. Efficacy of omega-3 in the treatment of polycystic ovary syndrome. J. Obstet. Gynaecol. 2013;33(3):289-291.

64. Feldeisen SE, Tucker KL. Nutritional strategies in the prevention and treatment of metabolic syndrome. Appl Physiol Nutr Metab. 2007;32(1):46-60.

65. Grundt JH, Nakling J, Eide GE, Markestad T. Possible relation between maternal consumption of added sugar and sugar-sweetened beverages and birth weight -- time trends in a population. BMC public health. 2012;12(1):901.

66. Borgen I, Aamodt G, Harsem N, Haugen M, Meltzer HM, Brantsaeter AL. Maternal sugar consumption and risk of preeclampsia in nulliparous Norwegian women. European journal of clinical nutrition. 2012;66(8):920-925.

67. NBJ's Supplement Business Report. Nutrition Business Journal;2012.

68. Wang Y, Storlien LH, Jenkins AB, et al. Dietary variables and glucose tolerance in pregnancy. Diabetes Care. 2000;23(4):460-464.

69. Bo S, Menato G, Lezo A, et al. Dietary fat and gestational hyperglycaemia. Diabetologia. 2001;44(8):972-978.

70. Radesky JS, Oken E, Rifas-Shiman SL, Kleinman KP, Rich-Edwards JW, Gillman MW. Diet during early pregnancy and development of gestational diabetes. Paediatric and perinatal epidemiology. 2008;22(1):47-59.

71. Hornstra G. Essential fatty acids in mothers and their neonates. The American journal of clinical nutrition. 2000;71(5 Suppl):1262S-1269S.

72. Dietary reference intakes for energy and the micronutrients, carbohydrates, fat, fiber and fatty acids. Washington, DC: National Academy Press; 2002.

73. Lauritzen L, Carlson SE. Maternal fatty acid status during pregnancy and lactation and relation to newborn and infant status. Maternal & child nutrition. 2011;7 Suppl 2:41-58.

74. Sanders TA. Essential fatty acid requirements of vegetarians in pregnancy, lactation, and infancy. The American journal of clinical nutrition. 1999;70(3 Suppl):555S-559S.

75. Ogle A. Before Your Pregnancy: a 90-day guide for couples on how to prepare for a healthy conception. New York, NY: Ballantine Books; 2011.

76. Carlson SE, Werkman SH, Tolley EA. Effect of long-chain n-3 fatty acid supplementation on visual acuity and growth of preterm infants with and without bronchopulmonary dysplasia. Am. J. Clin. Nutr. 1996;63(5):687-697.

77. Carlson SE, Colombo J, Gajewski BJ, et al. DHA supplementation and pregnancy outcomes. Am. J. Clin. Nutr. 2013.

78. Patrelli TS, Dall'asta A, Gizzo S, et al. Calcium supplementation and prevention of preeclampsia: a meta-analysis. J Maternal Fetal Neonatal Med. 2012;25(12):2570-2574.

79. Hofmeyr GJ, Lawrie TA, Atallah AN, Duley L. Calcium supplementation during pregnancy for preventing hypertensive disorders and related

problems. Cochrane Database Syst Rev. 2010(8):CD001059.

80. Dror DK, Allen LH. Interventions with vitamins B6, B12 and C in pregnancy. Paediatric and perinatal epidemiology. 2012;26 Suppl 1:55-74.

81. Rossi AC, Mullin PM. Prevention of pre-eclampsia with low-dose aspirin or vitamins C and E in women at high or low risk: a systematic review with meta-analysis. Euro J Obstetrics, gynecology, reprod bio. 2011;158(1):9-16.

82. Haugen M, Brantsaeter AL, Trogstad L, et al. Vitamin D supplementation and reduced risk of preeclampsia in nulliparous women. Epidemiology. 2009;20(5):720-726.

83. Foote J, Rengers B. Maternal use of herbal supplements. Nutrition in Complementary Care. 2000.

84. Cartwright, MM. Herbal use during pregnancy and lactation: a need for caution. The Digest 2001;(Summer):1-3. American Dietetic Association Public Health/Community Nutrition Practice Group.

85. Third Report of the National Cholesterol Education Program (NCEP) Expert Panel on Detection, Evaluation, and Treatment of High Blood Cholesterol in Adults (Adult Treatment Panel III) final report. Circulation. 2002;106(25):3143-3421.

86. Carmina E, Legro RS, Stamets K, Lowell J, Lobo RA. Difference in body weight between American and Italian women with polycystic ovary syndrome: influence of the diet. Hum. Reprod. 2003;18(11):2289-2293.

87. Vanky E, Nordskar JJ, Leithe H, Hjorth-Hansen AK, Martinussen M, Carlsen SM. Breast size increment during pregnancy and breastfeeding in mothers with polycystic ovary syndrome: a follow-up study of a randomised controlled trial on metformin versus placebo. BJOG. 2012;119(11):1403-1409.

88. Kris-Etherton PM, Harris WS, Appel LJ. Fish consumption, fish oil, omega-3 fatty acids, and cardiovascular disease. Arterioscler. Thromb. Vasc. Biol. 2003;23(2):e20-30.

89. Oh K, Hu FB, Manson JE, Stampfer MJ, Willett WC. Dietary fat intake and risk of coronary heart disease in women: 20 years of follow-up of the nurses' health study. Am. J. Epidemiol. 2005;161(7):672-679.

90. Gabbay MaK, H. Use of metformin to increase breastmilk production in women with insulin resistance: A case series. Presented at the Academy of Breastfeeding Medicine Conference; October 2003.

91. Hu FB, Bronner L, Willett WC, et al. Fish and omega-3 fatty acid intake and risk of coronary heart disease in women. JAMA. 2002;287(14):1815-1821.

92. Chavarro JE, Rich-Edwards JW, Rosner BA, Willett WC. Protein intake and ovulatory infertility. Am. J. Obstet. Gynecol. 2008;198(2):210 e211-217.

93. Chavarro JE, Rich-Edwards JW, Rosner BA, Willett WC. Dietary fatty acid intakes and the risk of ovulatory infertility. Am. J. Clin. Nutr. 2007;85(1):231-237.

94. Ornstein RM, Copperman NM, Jacobson MS. Effect of weight loss on menstrual function in adolescents with polycystic ovary syndrome. J. Pediatr. Adolesc. Gynecol. 2011;24(3):161-165.

95. Gannon MC, Nuttall FQ, Neil BJ, Westphal SA. The insulin and glucose responses to meals of glucose plus various proteins in type II diabetic subjects. Metabolism. 1988;37(11):1081-1088.

96. Feig DS, Briggs GG, Koren G. Oral antidiabetic agents in pregnancy and lactation: a paradigm shift? Annals of pharmacotherapy. 2007;41(7):1174-1180.

97. Glueck CJ, Wang P. Metformin before and during pregnancy and lactation in polycystic ovary syndrome. Expert opinion on drug safety. 2007;6(2):191-198.

98. Hubbard R, Kosch CL, Sanchez A, Sabate J, Berk L, Shavlik G. Effect of dietary protein on serum insulin and glucagon levels in hyper- and normocholesterolemic men. Atherosclerosis. 1989;76(1):55-61.

99. Linne Y, Dye L, Barkeling B, Rossner S. Long-term weight development in women: a 15-year follow-up of the effects of pregnancy. Obes Res. 2004;12(7):1166-1178.

100. Chavarro JE, Rich-Edwards JW, Rosner BA, Willett WC. A prospective study of dietary carbohydrate quantity and quality in relation to risk of ovulatory infertility. Eur. J. Clin. Nutr. 2009;63(1):78-86.

101. Danby FW. Nutrition and acne. Clin. Dermatol. 2010;28(6):598-604.

Chapter 6

PCOS AND AGING

Once referred to as the "medical black hole,"[1] the transition through menopause has been largely ignored in women with PCOS. The majority of studies on PCOS have examined the reproductive and metabolic disturbances of women of reproductive age, yet PCOS is a chronic condition that needs to be managed throughout a women's life.

Now that more is known about the syndrome and the influence of insulin on the increased risk of T2DM and CVD, changes in PCOS beyond the reproductive years is getting the attention they deserve.

Longitudinal studies have been conducted with postmenopausal women who were first studied 20 to 30 years ago to examine changes in PCOS presentation associated with age.[2-4] Several studies have tried to answer questions about PCOS and aging, such as: Does the syndrome get worse or does it improve after menopause? Can PCOS be "cured" or simply disappear?

The purpose of this chapter is to discuss the research that has been presented thus far regarding aging women with PCOS, including changes in hormones, body composition, and metabolic parameters, and to discuss the implications to patients and practice.

THE EFFECT OF AGE ON REPRODUCTIVE HORMONES

During the childbearing years, women with PCOS experience an imbalance in reproductive hormones; typically, androgens and LH levels are higher, whereas levels of FSH and SHBG are lower.

As women age and transition through menopause, estrogen levels naturally decrease. But what effect does aging and declining estrogen have on reproductive hormones for women with PCOS? According to the research thus far, it appears that sex hormones eventually ameliorate with age but remain different in women with PCOS than those without the syndrome.

In a prospective study, Schmidt et al reexamined 25 women with PCOS whom they first examined 21 years prior and matched them with non-PCOS women.[3] They found that total testosterone gradually decreased to normal age-related levels by age 61 and that DHEA, the precursor to testosterone, declines with age but does not reach normal levels until 20 years after menopause. Older women with PCOS had lower levels of SHBG, a hormone that binds to testosterone, and hyperandrogenicity, as expressed by higher free androgen index levels than controls. Lower levels of FSH also persisted after menopause.

Two cross-sectional studies compared postmenopausal women with PCOS in the sixth decade of life with non-PCOS women.[5,6] Markopoulos et al found that postmenopausal women with PCOS had significantly elevated androgen levels, including total testosterone, androstenedione, and DHEA, and increased levels of free androgen index, supporting the findings of Schmidt et al.[3,5] The latter researchers also reported that SHBG was significantly decreased compared with non-PCOS women.[3]

In the other cross-sectional study, Puurunen et al also found elevated androstenedione levels and lower SHBG in postmenopausal women with PCOS compared with control women.[6] Because SHBG binds to testosterone, a decline in SHBG will lead to hyperandrogenism with a greater amount of circulating androgens.

These studies indicate that hyperandrogensism persists beyond menopause in women with PCOS. This evidence, along with research that shows antimullerian hormone levels or the number of ovarian follicles are significantly higher in women with PCOS compared with controls,[7] led some researchers to conclude that women with PCOS reach menopause two[7] to five[3,5] years later than women without the syndrome. Tehrani et al, for example, found that while women without the syndrome reached menopause at the average age of 49, women with PCOS did not reach menopause until age 51.[7]

Numerous studies have demonstrated that women with PCOS experience improved menstrual regularity as they age.[2,3,8-10] Improvements regarding menstruation occurred with women in their early 30s,[8,9] suggesting that nonovulatory women with PCOS may have a better chance of conceiving as they get older.

There are several theories about why women with PCOS experience regular menstrual cycles as they age. Two are that androgen production by the adrenal glands decreases over time[11] or that less testosterone is released from fewer theca cells in the ovaries.[9]

Despite a decrease in overall androgen production with age, levels still remain elevated in postmenopausal women with PCOS.[8] Although older women with PCOS reported fewer hot flashes and episodes of sweating compared with women without PCOS, they also reported significantly more hirsutism compared with controls (64% vs. 9%) and more vaginal dryness.[3] Constant exposure to elevated androgens could have a lasting effect on excessive facial and body hair, hair loss, and even balding in women with PCOS that extends past menopause.[3]

"My biggest concern as I get older is that I will have a bald spot on my head just like my grandmother did." **Teresa, age 57**

Although symptoms may present differently, hirsutism can significantly impact body image and self-esteem, contributing to anxiety, depression, and overall poor quality of life in older women with PCOS.[12] It is not uncommon for older women with PCOS to indicate that they went from experiencing mild hirsutism prior to menopause to severe hirsutism afterward. One patient tearfully shared pictures of herself in her early 40s with a full head of hair only to have severe alopccia by the age of 67. Other women have experienced only slight hair growth on their face until menopause, when their facial hair became problematic.

BODY COMPOSITION CHANGES WITH AGE

"I'm past menopause, but I still look 5 months pregnant."
Lorraine, age 60

Women of all ages experience body composition changes as they age. In general, menopausal women are prone to rapid weight gain and increased visceral fat.[13] However, only a handful of studies have examined body composition and age in women with PCOS.

Schmidt and colleagues measured the height, weight, and waist circumference of women with PCOS ages 61 to 79 and found that as the women aged, they lost height and had greater waist-to-hip ratios.[3] The women also experienced greater increases in BMI, supporting findings of earlier research.[14,15] Age-related body fat redistribution along with height loss explained why women with PCOS had larger waist circumference measurements and increased BMI values as they got older.[3]

In their study, Carmina et al found that waist circumference progressively increased with age among all PCOS phenotype groups, becoming significant after 15 years.[2] Women with hyperandrogenism and anonovulation had a significantly higher BMI and waist circumference measurements compared with other PCOS phenotypes and control subjects. Interestingly, body weight did not significantly change during the 20-year follow-up, similar to the findings of Schmidt.[2]

Elevated waist circumference is associated with an increased risk of metabolic syndrome,[16-18] T2DM,[17] and CVD[19] in women with PCOS. In addition, increased waist circumference and BMI can negatively impact body image, possibly affecting self-esteem and increasing the risk of depression in this population.[20]

METABOIC CHANGES WITH AGE

While it appears that reproductive hormones in women with PCOS improve with age, the same is not true regarding metabolic abnormalities. Reproductive-age women with the syndrome have an increased risk of CVD[19] and T2DM[17,21,22] compared with non-PCOS women because of hyperinsulinemia, elevated CRP levels, and dyslipidemia.[21] Both the International Diabetes Federation and the American Diabetes Association recognize PCOS as a nonmodifiable risk factor for T2DM.[23,24] Several studies have shown that as women with PCOS age, their risk of CVD[6,14,25] and T2DM[4,6,14] increases, stressing the need for early detection and aggressive treatment of the syndrome.

CVD Risk

Puurunen et al found that postmenopausal women with PCOS had greater high-sensitivity CRP levels than women without PCOS and that these levels worsened with age.[6] Research also showed that as women with PCOS approach menopause, they have an increased prevalence of coronary artery calcification.[26]

In a study by Talbott et al, women with PCOS were compared with controls.[26] Sixty-three percent of the women with PCOS had coronary artery calcification compared with 42% of controls after adjusting for age and BMI.[26] African American women and women who had surgical menopause experienced the greatest effect as an independent risk factor for subclinical atherosclerosis when adjusted for age and BMI.[26]

Krentz et al found the risk of CVD is higher in postmenopausal white women with PCOS who did not have T2DM and who had intact ovaries.[25] They found that the prevalence of CVD was similar among women with PCOS who had hysterectomies than women without PCOS (27.3% vs. 24.4%).[25] It is not known, however, whether CVD risk is modified by surgical menopause in women with PCOS. Future studies in this area are warranted.

Research shows that lipid metabolism worsens as women with PCOS age, especially regarding triglyceride and HDL concentrations. While LDL cholesterol levels were found to be similar for middle-aged women with PCOS and controls, HDL was reduced and triglyceride levels were higher than controls.[25]

Marcut et al found deterioration in lipid metabolism between the third and fourth decade of life as they observed an increase in total cholesterol, LDL cholesterol, and triglycerides.[14] Only triglycerides correlated significantly with BMI among older women with PCOS (more than 30 years). These findings support those of other researchers who demonstrated an unfavorable lipid profile (elevated triglycerides and reduced HDL concentrations) in postmenopausal women with the syndrome.[15,25]

In a retrospective cohort study involving 2,301 women, Mani et al found that along with an increased prevalence of T2DM, women with PCOS had a higher incidence and age-specific prevalence of myocardial infarction and angina, with more than one-quarter of women older than 65 having experienced a myocardial infarction or angina.[22]

Glucose, Insulin Metabolism, and T2DM Risk

Limited data exist regarding insulin and glucose metabolism in postmenopausal women with PCOS. Women with PCOS who are obese have been shown to have a fivefold risk of developing T2DM compared with age- and weight-matched controls.[27] Macut et al showed the deterioration of glucose and insulin sensitivity related to age as BMI increased in women with PCOS.[14] In addition, women developed hyperinsulinemia and insulin resistance by the third decade of life.[14]

Puurunen et al demonstrated impaired glucose metabolism and increased insulin secretion after menopause in women with PCOS, independent of BMI.[6] Interestingly, there were more cases of IGT and T2DM among the women with PCOS. Carmina et al did not observe any significant changes in insulin or insulin resistance among patients with PCOS at their 20-year follow-up, although the average age was 42.[2]

In a retrospective longitudinal follow-up study, Brown et al examined patients with PCOS at an outpatient clinic on two different occasions.[8] They found that patients who had their follow-up visit six months to 3.9 years later showed a decrease in insulin resistance, whereas those who visited the clinic four to seven years later showed an increase in insulin resistance.[8] The difference in insulin resistance between the groups could be explained by the fact that patients may have been taking metformin or other insulin-sensitizing medications between visits or suggests the positive impact of lifestyle intervention.

At the clinic where patients were assessed, women were counseled in regard to lifestyle and exercise modification. As adjustments to lifestyle are difficult to sustain, those who had the shorter follow-up time may have improved their insulin sensitivity because of the support they received from counseling, whereas those who didn't follow up until much later had worse insulin resistance, perhaps because of the lack of support or the influence of aging.

Several studies have shown a significant trend toward an increasing prevalence of T2DM among aging women with PCOS. Women who had a greater waist circumference, BMI, or family history of diabetes had a higher prevalence of T2DM.[4,28] Gambineri et al showed the prevalence of T2DM in women with PCOS at middle age is 6.8 times higher than that of the general female population of similar age.[4] Furthermore, it has been suggested that there is a rapid progression from IGT to T2DM in women with PCOS[1,29] and that T2DM may occur earlier than expected in PCOS compared with the general population.[4]

For this reason, the Androgen Excess and PCOS Society[29] recommends screening for IGT and T2DM with a two-hour OGTT every two years in women with PCOS who have normal glucose levels and annually in those with elevated glucose levels.

Boudreaux et al found that obese women with PCOS had a fivefold increased risk of developing T2DM compared with age-adjusted controls, indicating that BMI and obesity may be important factors in the development of T2DM in women with PCOS.[4,27] Interestingly, the study by Gambineri et al also showed the risk of developing T2DM decreased as SHBG increased.[4] It is believed that SHBG and hyperandrogenemia may influence the development of underlying metabolic dysfunction, glucose intolerance, and T2DM[4,30] and that high levels of SHBG may protect against T2DM.[30]

MNT FOR OLDER WOMEN WITH PCOS

Clearly, women with PCOS face life-long health risks extending beyond the reproductive years. Talbott et al stated that "the menopause transition along with life-long increases in cardiovascular risk factors (obesity, hyperinsulinemia, increased LDL, and decreased HDL) continues to create an adverse environment and a process in women with PCOS that outpaces those of non-PCOS women."[26]

As discussed in Chapter 2, evidence-based information regarding nutrition management for PCOS does not lend itself to a definitive treatment plan and is based mostly on women of reproductive age. Evidence of nutrition management for older women with the disease is scant.

Weight loss of 5% to 10% of total body weight has been shown to improve both reproductive and metabolic parameters associated with PCOS.[31-34] It then can be assumed that weight loss will improve metabolic parameters in older women with PCOS as well.

Berrino et al found a significant increase in SHBG and decrease in serum testosterone levels along with decreases in waist-to-hip ratio, total cholesterol, and fasting glucose concentrations in postmenopausal hyperandrogenic women who received an ad libitum diet that was low in animal fats and refined carbohydrates and high in low-GI foods, monounsaturated and omega-3 fatty acids, and phytoestrogens.[35] In a small sample size of women with PCOS ages 18 to 45, a hypocaloric diet supplemented with protein reduced body weight, fat mass, and serum cholesterol more than a diet supplemented with simple sugars.[36]

A range of potential dietary approaches have shown favorable effects on weight loss and metabolic parameters in PCOS, including modifying GI and GL, carbohydrate, fat, or protein or using meal replacements. While there is no conclusive evidence of one dietary strategy being superior to another in achieving long-term weight loss and metabolic improvement, what is clear is that older women with PCOS require aggressive MNT interventions to prevent or improve metabolic abnormalities and reduce risk for disease.

Because of increased CRP levels as people age, older women with PCOS may benefit from a diet that emphasizes anti-inflammatory foods, including fiber, red wine, and omega-3 fatty acids.[37] Certainly, studies examining at the optimal diet composition for older women are needed.

Barriers to Nutrition Counseling and Weight Management

"I've been on so many diets, all with different rules, that I don't know what to eat anymore." Jane, age 53

Dietitians may find unique challenges when counseling older women with PCOS. Older women with PCOS who have struggled with their weight for most of their lives may be chronic dieters, having followed numerous diets in the past. As a result, they may distrust their ability to self-regulate food intake and engage in distorted eating practices, including restricting, bingeing, purging, using diet pills and laxatives, or excessively exercising, potentially adding to the pathogenesis of PCOS.[13,38] Women with PCOS may also hold negative and false food beliefs that need to be addressed in nutrition sessions.

There are several physiological factors that may pose specific barriers to weight management in the PCOS population. Since insulin is a growth hormone, hyperinsulinemia or insulin resistance may predispose women with PCOS to gain weight or make losing weight more of a challenge.[13] Older women with PCOS may find it particularly difficult to manage insulin levels and lose weight than younger women with the disease, as insulin levels have been shown to worsen with age.[6,14]

Also, elevated androgens contribute to fat storage and contribute to insulin resistance.[13] Weight-loss studies have shown higher drop-out rates among women with PCOS (26% to 38%) compared with women without PCOS,[13] perhaps related to the weight management challenges of excess insulin and androgens. In addition, it has been suggested that women with PCOS have impaired appetite regulation, with abnormal levels of ghrelin[39,40] and CCK,[41] posing additional weight management challenges.

Brown et al implied the positive impact of lifestyle counseling for improving insulin sensitivity in older women with PCOS.[8] Therefore, dietitians can provide nutrition counseling and education to older women with PCOS to help them make positive changes to their eating habits to improve their health and reduce disease risk.

In summary, PCOS does not simply disappear as women get older, and women with PCOS differ in reproductive hormones past menopause. Most importantly, inflammatory and metabolic parameters worsen with age, putting women with PCOS at increased risk of life-long health issues beyond menopause, especially the risk of developing CVD and T2DM.

The nutrition management for older women with PCOS should take into account the risk of long-term complications associated with the disease. This supports the need for effective and aggressive treatment involving diet, lifestyle, and insulin sensitizers for older women with PCOS who have metabolic complications. Early detection and proactive treatment of PCOS are crucial to prevent the long-term metabolic consequences associated with this complex syndrome.

FUTURE IMPLICATIONS

We are only beginning to understand how PCOS changes with age. The studies presented here have increased the knowledge and understanding of the physiological changes in women with PCOS past menopause compared with their non-PCOS peers. However, there is still much to learn regarding how diet, supplements, medications, physical activity, and lifestyle changes affect women with PCOS as they grow older and whether changes to these areas can improve or even prevent the worsening of metabolic parameters.

In addition to the need for further research to confirm the evidence discussed in this chapter, numerous questions remain, such as the following: What role do androgens play in the pathogenesis of CVD? How does pregnancy and breast-feeding affect the natural evolution of PCOS over time? Do some PCOS phenotypes fair better with age than others?

CHAPTER SUMMARY

- Women with PCOS differ in reproductive hormones after menopause.
- Postmenopausal women with PCOS are exposed to higher adrenal and ovarian androgen levels than women without PCOS.
- The reproductive life span of PCOS extends beyond that of non-PCOS women.
- Women with PCOS experience regular menstrual cycles with age.
- CRP levels, impaired glucose metabolism, and insulin resistance worsen after menopause.
- Waist circumference increases with age in women with PCOS.
- Women with PCOS can experience life-long health issues beyond menopause.
- Aggressive treatment with diet and lifestyle modification is needed for this population.

REFERENCES

1. Fenton A, Panay N. Management of polycystic ovary syndrome in postmenopausal women: a medical black hole. Climacteric. 2008;11(2):89-90.
2. Carmina E, Campagna AM, Lobo RA. A 20-year follow-up of young women with polycystic ovary syndrome. Obstet. Gynecol. 2012;119(2 Pt 1):263-269.
3. Schmidt J, Brannstrom M, Landin-Wilhelmsen K, Dahlgren E. Reproductive hormone levels and anthropometry in postmenopausal women with polycystic ovary syndrome (PCOS): a 21-year follow-up study of women diagnosed with PCOS around 50 years ago and their age-matched controls. J. Clin. Endocrinol. Metab. 2011;96(7):2178-2185.
4. Gambineri A, Patton L, Altieri P, et al. Polycystic Ovary Syndrome Is a Risk Factor for Type 2 Diabetes: Results From a Long-Term Prospective Study. Diabetes. 2012.
5. Markopoulos MC, Rizos D, Valsamakis G, et al. Hyperandrogenism in women with polycystic ovary syndrome persists after menopause. J. Clin. Endocrinol. Metab. 2011;96(3):623-631.
6. Puurunen J, Piltonen T, Morin-Papunen L, et al. Unfavorable hormonal, metabolic, and inflammatory alterations persist after menopause in women with PCOS. J. Clin. Endocrinol. Metab. 2011;96(6):1827-1834.
7. Tehrani FR, Solaymani-Dodaran M, Hedayati M, Azizi F. Is polycystic ovary syndrome an exception for reproductive aging? Hum. Reprod. 2010;25(7):1775-1781.
8. Brown ZA, Louwers YV, Fong SL, et al. The phenotype of polycystic ovary syndrome ameliorates with aging. Fertil. Steril. 2011;96(5):1259-1265.
9. Elting MW, Korsen TJ, Rekers-Mombarg LT, Schoemaker J. Women with polycystic ovary syndrome gain regular menstrual cycles when ageing. Hum. Reprod. 2000;15(1):24-28.
10. Winters SJ, Talbott E, Guzick DS, Zborowski J, McHugh KP. Serum testosterone levels decrease in middle age in women with the polycystic ovary syndrome. Fertil. Steril. 2000;73(4):724-729.
11. Bili H, Laven J, Imani B, Eijkemans MJ, Fauser BC. Age-related differences in features associated with polycystic ovary syndrome in normogonadotrophic oligo-amenorrhoeic infertile women of reproductive years. Eur. J. Endocrinol. 2001;145(6):749-755.
12. de Niet JE, de Koning CM, Pastoor H, et al. Psychological well-being and sexarche in women with polycystic ovary syndrome. Hum. Reprod. 2010;25(6):1497-1503.

13. Moran LJ, Lombard CB, Lim S, Noakes M, Teede HJ. Polycystic ovary syndrome and weight management. Womens Health. 2010;6(2):271-283.

14. Macut D, Micic D, Parapid B, et al. Age and body mass related changes of cardiovascular risk factors in women with polycystic ovary syndrome. Vojnosanit. Pregl. 2002;59(6):593-599.

15. Margolin E, Zhornitzki T, Kopernik G, Kogan S, Schattner A, Knobler H. Polycystic ovary syndrome in post-menopausal women--marker of the metabolic syndrome. Maturitas. 2005;50(4):331-336.

16. Hudecova M, Holte J, Olovsson M, Larsson A, Berne C, Sundstrom-Poromaa I. Prevalence of the metabolic syndrome in women with a previous diagnosis of polycystic ovary syndrome: long-term follow-up. Fertil. Steril. 2011;96(5):1271-1274.

17. Moran LJ, Misso ML, Wild RA, Norman RJ. Impaired glucose tolerance, type 2 diabetes and metabolic syndrome in polycystic ovary syndrome: a systematic review and meta-analysis. Hum. Reprod. Update. 2010;16(4):347-363.

18. Ehrmann DA, Liljenquist DR, Kasza K, Azziz R, Legro RS, Ghazzi MN. Prevalence and predictors of the metabolic syndrome in women with polycystic ovary syndrome. J. Clin. Endocrinol. Metab. 2006;91(1):48-53.

19. Cascella T, Palomba S, De Sio I, et al. Visceral fat is associated with cardiovascular risk in women with polycystic ovary syndrome. Hum. Reprod. 2008;23(1):153-159.

20. Cipkala-Gaffin J, Talbott EO, Song MK, Bromberger J, Wilson J. Associations between psychologic symptoms and life satisfaction in women with polycystic ovary syndrome. J Womens Health. 2012;21(2):179-187.

21. Tomlinson J, Millward A, Stenhouse E, Pinkney J. Type 2 diabetes and cardiovascular disease in polycystic ovary syndrome: what are the risks and can they be reduced? Diabet. Med. 2010;27(5):498-515.

22. Mani H, Levy MJ, Davies MJ, et al. Diabetes and cardiovascular events in women with polycystic ovary syndrome; a 20 years retrospective cohort study. Clin. Endocrinol. 2012.

23. Alberti KG, Zimmet P, Shaw J. International Diabetes Federation: a consensus on Type 2 diabetes prevention. Diabet. Med. 2007;24(5):451-463.

24. Association AD. Screening for type 2 diabetes. Diabetes Care. 2004;27:11-14.

25. Krentz AJ, von Muhlen D, Barrett-Connor E. Searching for polycystic ovary syndrome in postmenopausal women: evidence of a dose-effect association with prevalent cardiovascular disease. Menopause. 2007;14(2):284-292.

26. Talbott EO, Zborowski J, Rager J, Stragand JR. Is there an independent effect of polycystic ovary syndrome (PCOS) and menopause on the

prevalence of subclinical atherosclerosis in middle aged women? Vasc Health Risk Manag. 2008;4(2):453-462.

27. Boudreaux MY, Talbott EO, Kip KE, Brooks MM, Witchel SF. Risk of T2DM and impaired fasting glucose among PCOS subjects: results of an 8-year follow-up. Curr Diab Rep. 2006;6(1):77-83.

28. Dabadghao P, Roberts BJ, Wang J, Davies MJ, Norman RJ. Glucose tolerance abnormalities in Australian women with polycystic ovary syndrome. Med. J. Aust. 2007;187(6):328-331.

29. Salley KE, Wickham EP, Cheang KI, Essah PA, Karjane NW, Nestler JE. Glucose intolerance in polycystic ovary syndrome--a position statement of the Androgen Excess Society. J. Clin. Endocrinol. Metab. 2007;92(12):4546-4556.

30. Ding EL, Song Y, Manson JE, Rifai N, Buring JE, Liu S. Plasma sex steroid hormones and risk of developing type 2 diabetes in women: a prospective study. Diabetologia. 2007;50(10):2076-2084.

31. Moran LJ, Pasquali R, Teede HJ, Hoeger KM, Norman RJ. Treatment of obesity in polycystic ovary syndrome: a position statement of the Androgen Excess and Polycystic Ovary Syndrome Society. Fertil. Steril. 2009;92(6):1966-1982.

32. Thomson RL, Buckley JD, Noakes M, Clifton PM, Norman RJ, Brinkworth GD. The effect of a hypocaloric diet with and without exercise training on body composition, cardiometabolic risk profile, and reproductive function in overweight and obese women with polycystic ovary syndrome. J. Clin. Endocrinol. Metab. 2008;93(9):3373-3380.

33. Clark AM, Ledger W, Galletly C, et al. Weight loss results in significant improvement in pregnancy and ovulation rates in anovulatory obese women. Hum. Reprod. 1995;10(10):2705-2712.

34. Hoeger KM, Kochman L, Wixom N, Craig K, Miller RK, Guzick DS. A randomized, 48-week, placebo-controlled trial of intensive lifestyle modification and/or metformin therapy in overweight women with polycystic ovary syndrome: a pilot study. Fertil. Steril. 2004;82(2):421-429.

35. Berrino F, Bellati C, Secreto G, et al. Reducing bioavailable sex hormones through a comprehensive change in diet: the diet and androgens (DIANA) randomized trial. Cancer Epidemiol. Biomarkers Prev. 2001;10(1):25-33.

36. Kasim-Karakas SE, Cunningham WM, Tsodikov A. Relation of nutrients and hormones in polycystic ovary syndrome. Am. J. Clin. Nutr. 2007;85(3):688-694.

37. Liepa GU, Sengupta A, Karsies D. Polycystic ovary syndrome (PCOS) and other androgen excess-related conditions: can changes in dietary intake make a difference? Nutr. Clin. Pract. 2008;23(1):63-71.

38. Michelmore KF, Balen AH, Dunger DB. Polycystic ovaries and eating disorders: Are they related? Hum. Reprod. 2001;16(4):765-769.

39. Krentz AJ, Barrett-Connor E. Reduced serum ghrelin in a putative postmenopausal polycystic ovary syndrome phenotype. Fertil. Steril. 2009;92(5):1753-1754.

40. Panidis D, Asteriadis C, Georgopoulos NA, et al. Decreased active, total and altered active to total ghrelin ratio in normal weight women with the more severe form of polycystic ovary syndrome. Eur. J. Obstet. Gynecol. Reprod. Biol. 2010;149(2):170-174.

41. Hirschberg AL, Naessen S, Stridsberg M, Bystrom B, Holtet J. Impaired cholecystokinin secretion and disturbed appetite regulation in women with polycystic ovary syndrome. Gynecol. Endocrinol. 2004;19(2):79-87.

Chapter 7

PSYCHOLOGICAL ASPECTS OF PCOS

By Stephanie B. Mattei, PsyD,
And
Michelle Shwarz, MSEd

Julie is 13. She began menstruating two years ago but without regularity. Recently, Julie has noticed her body changing in ways that are different from her friends. She worries about the extra hair sprouting on her chest, belly, and face. She is covered in acne and a bit concerned that she is somewhat heavier than her peers.

Embarrassed, Julie asks her mother to take her to the doctor. Her mother tells her that she will grow out of these problems and believes that Julie is experiencing normal adolescent worries about her developing body.

In the meantime, Julie starts waxing the unwanted hair and secretly starts skipping breakfast and lunch in the hopes that her belly will "go away." She struggles to concentrate and focus on her schoolwork. All she can think about is how "weird" she looks and feels. She is consumed by her thoughts and finds solace only when she is alone in her room.

At 15, Julie still gets her period irregularly—twice a year at most with heavy monthly spotting. This irregularity causes additional anxiety since she never knows when she will get her period or when the spotting will just "show up."

Additionally, Julie continues to gain weight. Her fasting diet has slipped into a fasting/binging cycle, which contributes to feelings of guilt and shame, and thoughts that she is inferior to her peers who are thinner.

Finally, Julie convinces her mother to take her to the doctor, who subsequently tells Julie to stop eating junk food because she is obese and prescribes birth control pills. Resentful of the doctor's diet advice but relieved to get some hope of normalcy, Julie starts taking the birth control and finally gets her monthly period with extreme predictability plus her acne virtually clears up.

Julie and her mother often have conversations about her stopping the birth control because her mother secretly fears that Julie now has permission to have sex. This strains their relationship, and Julie feels even more isolated. Julie's family, who were once the source of support, are now the source of even more stress.

Julie is cranky and irritable most of the time, but her mother again brushes it off as normal teenage behavior.

In addition, Julie continues to gain weight, sometimes 10 lbs in a month. In one year, Julie had gone from 180 lbs and a size 14 to 260 lbs and a size 22. She is devastated that she no longer can shop at the trendy stores where her girlfriends are getting their cute clothes. She starts losing her confidence that she will ever have the opportunity to date while in high school, let alone be in an intimate relationship or have sex. Julie begins defining herself by her low self-esteem.

Julie becomes depressed. She withdraws from her peer group and no longer participates in her favorite activities. Eating and sleeping become her primary activities out of school.

Julie is now 32 and met the love of her life seven years ago. During the past 17 years, Julie has cycled in and out of her depression. Her weight has fluctuated by 50 lbs or more per year, but she is acne free and gets her period every month because she is still taking birth control. She has been unsuccessful with sustained weight loss despite her diet and exercise efforts.

Julie and her husband have decided to start a family, and for the first time in nearly 20 years, she stops taking birth control. After the first few months without birth control, Julie does not get her period and excitedly takes a pregnancy test but receives a negative result. After two weeks, she still does not get her period and retakes the home test again with another negative result.

After trying for six months to become pregnant, Julie finally confides in her husband that she has not had her period the entire time. Her mood shifts from depressed to irritable. She is angry and frustrated more days than not.

Frustrated, Julie and her husband consult a fertility specialist. After taking a full history, the doctor performs an intravaginal ultrasound, confirming the presence of ovarian cysts. He diagnoses Julie as having PCOS.

While the physical symptoms of PCOS are becoming increasingly recognized in the medical world, knowledge about the psychological effects are lagging. In a study involving 72 women with PCOS, 57% presented with at least one psychiatric diagnosis.[1]

This chapter discusses the various psychological issues women with PCOS may experience. Issues about body image and self-esteem arise from abnormal stress responses that correlate with significant weight gain: hirsutism, acne, infertility, and issues with sex drive. Eating disorders, depression, anxiety, and bipolar disorder are also common clinical conditions observed in these women. Recommendations for treatment and appropriate professional referrals will help dietitians notice when an issue has arisen.

BODY IMAGE AND SELF-ESTEEM

"Nothing I do works. I watch my diet and exercise, yet I can't lose weight. I feel like a failure." **Serena, age 24**

Much like Julie, women with PCOS may feel ashamed about their body and the various symptoms they experience. They may feel ashamed that they cannot control their weight through exercise or diet, or are embarrassed about their dermatological symptoms, such as unwanted hair growth, acne, or balding.

Many physicians and health care professionals still lack enough education about the complexities of PCOS and, as a result, they may give supportive advice to their PCOS patients, such as to lose weight or don't worry, which only contributes to the urge to isolate themselves and avoid coping with the effects of the syndrome.

Most women in American society correlate their body image with self-esteem. Ironically, a person's actual size or appearance may not directly correlate with body image. Someone who is perceived as unattractive by others may have a positive body image, whereas someone who is perceived as attractive by others may have negative self-image.

Self-image is a valuation that someone places on herself and what she has to offer. It encompasses more than just body image; it may include perceived intelligence, kindness, altruism, and personality, all of which play a part in shaping self-image. Women with PCOS may overlook these aspects of self-image and consider their appearance to be more important in forming their self-image. They may desire a particular body shape or size and experience certain emotions about their ability to achieve it.

Research has shown that women with PCOS experience more body dissatisfaction and depression compared with their non-PCOS counterparts[2-5] as well as lowered quality of life.[6,7] Weight had the biggest negative impact on quality of life.[6] The majority of women with PCOS are overweight or obese, and it's not uncommon for them to be frustrated by unsuccessful weight-loss attempts and lack self-esteem. Additionally, the classic android body composition women with PCOS exhibit does not conform to society's ideal of thinness and can negatively impact body image.

Himelein and Thatcher suggested that "it may be more important for women with PCOS to improve body image rather than lose weight; body satisfaction may reduce emotional distress, whereas unsuccessful dieting might only increase it."[3] They also suggested that health care professionals be sensitive to the multiple complexities among body dissatisfaction, dieting, and depression when encouraging their patients to lose weight.[3]

STRESS RESPONSES AND WEIGHT

"Eating food is the only way to calm me down. But then after I eat, I feel incredibly guilty and more anxious." **Sara, age 29**

Stress is a given in the complicated lives of women today, and there has been a plethora of research regarding the impact stress has on humans. Americans engage in numerous unhealthful behaviors as a way of self-soothing, including comfort eating, poor diet choices, smoking, and inactivity. People experiencing stress are more likely to report anxiety or depression, and chronic stress increases the risk of obesity and chronic diseases.[8,9]

For women with PCOS, there is even more to deal with. Not only is there the typical stress reaction, but there may be additional responses because of the condition's hormonal impact.

Stress and depression stimulate hypothalamic-pituitary-adrenal axis activity.[10] A study done by Rutledge and Linden showed that women who are restrictive eaters tended to increase their food consumption under stress as opposed to nonrestrictive eaters.[11] In their review, Moore et al showed that higher stress resulted in less healthful dietary behaviors and higher body weight.[12]

In addition, because of the potential amplified physiological effect of stress on women with PCOS, the stress-eat reaction may last longer than for women without the diagnosis. Epel et al studied 59 healthy premenopausal women to determine the effect stress had on eating behaviors.[13] The women were observed in both stressful and controlled conditions. The research found that women who were stressed and had higher cortisol levels also had a higher caloric intake as opposed to those with lower cortisol levels who had lower caloric intake.

Interestingly, during the nonstress condition, both groups ate similar amounts. Additionally, the higher-cortisol group ate more sweet foods than did the lower-cortisol group. Another interesting finding is that a more negative mood in response to the stressors were significantly related to greater food consumption.[13]

These findings suggest that stress and increased eating behavior may be part of a vicious perpetual cycle that may be difficult for women with PCOS to combat because they produce more cortisol when repeatedly being stressed.[14,15] Excess cortisol contributes to increased visceral fat,[10,16] and women with PCOS have more visceral fat than normal women. Therefore, stress-reduction interventions for women with PCOS are recommended as part of treatment.[15]

HIRSUTISM AND DERMATOLOGICAL ISSUES

"To avoid having a dark shadow on my wedding day, I spent over an hour plucking each hair on my face the night before." **Katie, age 32**

Dermatological symptoms (e.g., acne, hirsutism, alopecia) significantly contribute to increased emotional disturbances for women with PCOS. Women are likely to see themselves as unfeminine or even monstrous.

According to Brady et al, excess facial hair is one of the most disturbing aspects of PCOS and causes women to spend a considerable amount of time and energy on hiding excessive hair growth.[2] Lipton et al studied 88 women with facial hair and found that 67% continually checked themselves in the mirror, with 76% of them checking with touch.[17] On average, these women spent 104 minutes per week managing unwanted hair.

Being overly concerned with appearance at any age can be problematic, but teens and young women especially have the added worry of being concerned with how others see them. This preoccupation with being "normal" or "pretty" not only contributes to negative body image but also influences the manner in which these girls and women interact with their environment. These women might be shy in social environments, isolate themselves, or even develop anxiety related to social events.

IRREGULAR MENSES, SEX DRIVE, AND INFERTILITY

"My biggest failure in life, without a doubt, has been my inability to have children." **Dawn, age 48**

Irregular menses, unusual sex drive, and issues with fertility can also contribute to low self-esteem.[2,18] With minimal education concerning the detection and diagnosis of PCOS, young women with irregular menstrual cycles often are left feeling confused and scared. Much like we saw with Julie, they do not understand what is happening to their bodies or why their periods are heavy, abnormal, or nonexistent or, more importantly, why this is happening to them. Consequently, life-long feelings of shame, frustration, failure, and guilt can lead to the reduced self-esteem that impacts body image.

Women with PCOS also experience issues with sex drive. Trent et al studied sexual behavior in adolescent girls with PCOS and discovered that these girls engaged in sexual relationships later than their non-PCOS counterparts.[19] Himelein and Thatcher hypothesized that this may be due to their perceived lack of sexual desirability.[3]

When this trend was investigated, a strong correlation among perceived sexual attraction, body image, and sexual satisfaction was found. Women with PCOS believed that their sexual partners weren't as satisfied with them as did women without PCOS.[20] Hirsutism, acne, and other factors were also linked to sexual satisfaction and social outgoingness.

It has been hypothesized that women diagnosed with PCOS have a higher sexual desire than other women because of the increase in male hormones. Several studies have dispelled this belief and have showed that women with PCOS experienced decrease sexual desire and perceived sexual attractiveness; libido did not correlate with androgen levels.[20,21]

Infertility, the most common medical complication associated with PCOS, occurs in approximately 75% of women who have been diagnosed with the syndrome because of anovulation.[22] The feelings of loss, grief, depression, and even anxiety that come with the desire to become pregnant and the inability to do so can be devastating. Women who experience this often ruminate on their infertility issues and have difficulty concentrating or thinking about anything else. Additionally, symptoms of depression such as anhedonia (diminished pleasure in activities that were once enjoyable), social isolation, or even thoughts about death or suicide may occur.

Left untreated, the impact of infertility can lead to debilitating dysfunction in women diagnosed with PCOS and the destruction of even the best intimate relationships. Conversely, mood disorders may exacerbate hormonal disturbances and affect infertility treatment.[10]

CLINICAL CONDITIONS

Women with PCOS also may suffer with clinical conditions that need to be treated with the assistance of a mental health professional, including binge-eating disorder (BED), bulimia, major depressive disorder, bipolar disorder, and anxiety.

As a dietitian, if you suspect that a patient may be suffering from one of these conditions, you need to get the opinion of a psychiatrist, psychologist, or other mental health professional to reach an appropriate diagnosis. These conditions, which can be treated successfully with empirically supported treatments, should be approached by the entire clinical treatment team as significant.[23,24]

BED and Bulimia Nervosa

According to the American Psychiatric Association, BED includes "recurrent episodes of binge eating that must occur, on average at least once per week for three months and be accompanied by a sense of lack of control with the absence of the regular use of inappropriate compensatory behaviors (such as self-induced vomiting, misuse of laxatives and other medications, fasting, and excessive exercises) that are characteristics of bulimia nervosa."[26]

As for prevalence, the DSM-5 indicates that 1.6% of females and .8% of males have BED."[26] Other sources indicate that BED occurs in 2% of the population.[27] Of importance is that while the nonpatient prevalence is small, the percentage of patients with BED seen by a dietitian is much higher, as it falls within the range of those patients seeking assistance for weight issues.

Bulimia nervosa is another eating disorder often found in women diagnosed with PCOS. It is categorized by binge eating and inappropriate compensatory methods to prevent weight gain.[26] Figure 7.1 shows the process of differentiating between BED and bulimia.[27] The major difference is the compensatory behavior that occurs in those with bulimia after a binge.

These patients frequently experience a mood disorder along with BED or bulimia. Often the mood disorder develops after the initial diagnosis of bulimia. Empirically supported treatments for BED and bulimia, such as cognitive behavioral therapy (CBT) and interpersonal therapy,[23,24] can assist patients in the recovery process. More information on the connection between PCOS and eating disorders can be found in Chapter 8.

Major Depression

Depression is a distinct psychological disorder that is different than the "blues" or "feeling down." It is also different from a grief response that may result from the death of a loved one or the end of a relationship. Depression depletes energy and interest in activities that once were pleasurable, and can recur throughout an individual's life.

Major depression disorder is diagnosed when an individual experiences one or more major depressive episodes without a history of manic, mixed, or hypomanic episodes. The individual must have experienced a significant change in functioning, where one of the major clinical manifestations is either depressed mood or loss of interest of pleasure. For a major depressive episode to be diagnosed, at least five of the following symptoms need to be present during a two-week period:

- Depressed mood most of the day nearly every day as indicated by either subjective report (e.g., feels sad or empty) or observation made by others (e.g., appears tearful). Note: In children and adolescents, this can be irritable mood.

Figure 7.1: BED and Bulimia Nervosa Diagnostic Flow Chart[27]

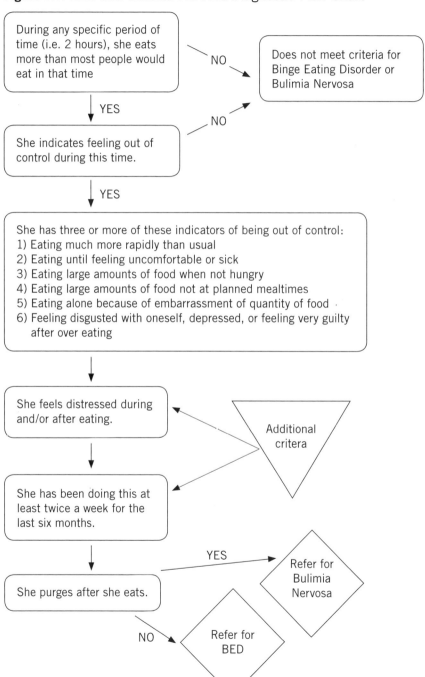

- Markedly diminished interest or pleasure in all, or almost all, activities most of the day nearly every day (as indicated by either subjective account or observation made by others).
- Significant weight loss when not dieting, weight gain (e.g., a change of more than 5% of body weight in a month), or a decrease or increase in appetite nearly every day. Note: In children, consider failure to make expected weight gains.
- Insomnia or hypersomnia nearly every day.
- Psychomotor agitation or retardation nearly every day (observable by others; not merely subjective feelings of restlessness or being slowed down).
- Fatigue or loss of energy every day.
- Feelings of worthlessness or excessive or inappropriate guilt (which may be delusional) nearly every day (not merely self-reproach or guilt about being sick).
- Diminished ability to think or concentrate or indecisiveness nearly every day (either by subjective account or as observed by others).
- Recurrent thoughts of death (not just fear of dying), recurrent suicidal ideation without a specific plan, or a suicide attempt with a specific plan.

Differentiating depression from other diagnoses as well as noting areas in the individual's life that have been impaired is important to the diagnosis. It is important for the dietitian to note that patients who experience depression will often report feeling sad, down, tearful, and generally unhappy.[26]

The relationship between major depression disorder and PCOS is well documented.[3,4,25] Prevalence rates of depressive symptoms in women with PCOS have been reported as high as 40%.[28] One study showed that suicide rates were seven times more common among women with PCOS.[29] A study published in the *Journal of Women's Health* found that women with PCOS who were heavier and had more children and less education had the greatest risk of depressive symptoms.[5]

An increase in insulin resistance has been associated with depression. Insulin also affects serotonin, a neurotransmitter that plays an important role in depression, aggression, anger, sexuality, body temperature, and appetite; disregulated serotonin is a leading cause in depression.[25] Brown reviewed the literature concerning the comorbid occurrence of insulin-resistant disorders such as diabetes and depression to strengthen the hypothesis that insulin resistance can cause depression in women with PCOS.[30] She pointed to a study that showed improvements in insulin sensitivity when non–insulin-resistant depressed patients were treated with antidepressants.[31] This study encouraged longer and larger-scale studies of comorbid depression and insulin sensitivity disorders to better understand this relationship.[32]

While the insulin resistance hypothesis regarding depression in women with PCOS is strong, it excludes lean women diagnosed with PCOS and those without insulin resistance. Keegan et al examined depression symptoms in lean PCOS patients with hirsutism.[33] They found a strong presence of depression in these women, which was higher than the comparison group of patients with cancer. Weight-matched controlled studies have shown a continued increased prevalence of depression in women with PCOS compared with normal controls, regardless of whether the women were lean or obese.[3,4]

There are additional hypotheses about the origins of depression in women with PCOS. Weiner et al compared mood states between women with PCOS and those with normal menstruation patterns.[34] They found a relationship between free testosterone and depression in women with PCOS experiencing more acute and long-standing depressive symptoms than women with normal hormone levels. In addition, other mood state differences, including hostility and anxiety, were linked to increased free testosterone in women diagnosed with PCOS.[34]

Bipolar Disorders

Bipolar I disorder, once called manic depression, is diagnosed when a client has a history of both depressive and manic episodes. Seeking pleasure, enjoying fast-paced activities, and exhibiting an increased rate of speech typically characterize the disorder. An individual can be diagnosed with bipolar I when she has experienced at least one manic episode or mixed episodes. While individuals may also have experienced a major depressive episode, its presence is not necessary for the diagnosis.

A manic episode is characterized by a distinct period of time (at least one week) in which there is an abnormally and persistently elevated expansive or irritated mood.[26] At least three or more of the following symptoms must also accompany the mood disturbance:

- Inflated self-esteem or grandiosity
- Decreased need for sleep (e.g., feels rested after only three hours of sleep)
- More talkative than usual or pressure to keep talking
- Flight of ideas of subjective experience that thoughts are racing
- Easily distracted, especially by unimportant or irrelevant external stimuli
- Increase in goal-directed activity (either socially, professionally, or sexually) or psychomotor agitation
- Excessive involvement in pleasurable activities that have a high potential for painful consequences (e.g., unrestrained buying sprees, sexual indiscretions, foolish business investments)

Another form of the disorder, Bipolar II, differs from bipolar I in that the patient has a history of at least one hypomanic episode. The symptoms of hypomanic episodes are similar to those of mania with differences in severity, degree of impairment as well as duration of the episode. In hypomania the symptoms last for at least four consecutive days, nearly every day.[26] Irritability is also more likely to be the key mood during hypomania rather than elevated mood, and the disturbance is not severe enough to cause marked impairment. That is, during a hypomanic episode, there would be no need for hospitalization.

If you suspect that a client may have a bipolar disorder, it is important to refer her to a mental health specialist for an appropriate assessment and diagnosis. Bipolar disorder is often diagnosed over a period of time after evaluating a personal and family history as well as observing symptoms.

During a consultation, you may notice a patient having a manic or hypomanic episode. Her rate of speech may increase; she may interrupt you frequently; or you may have difficulty getting her to stop talking. When she does talk, they may be in non sequiturs. That is, she may bounce from topic to topic without a logical progression of thoughts, and the episode may seem quite tangential.

Keeping her attention could be more difficult or you may find her focusing on details that are irrelevant. She may tell you about new plans unrelated to your counseling, such as new business ventures, having children, or starting or ending relationships.

Finally, her pleasure-seeking behavior is significantly different than that of people without bipolar disorder. The behaviors she engages in may have serious consequences, such as going on a spending spree, engaging in promiscuous sex, or suddenly quitting her job.

While these symptoms describe more of the clichéd manic episode, mania may present differently in women with PCOS. Particularly, where elevated mood, grandiosity, and hyperactivity may be the most notable symptoms of the aforementioned form of mania, women diagnosed with PCOS may present with irritability instead of elevated mood as the main feature of their mania.

As a dietitian working with women with PCOS, it is likely that you will come across a patient with bipolar disorder because of the high correlation between the two diagnoses. While there are numerous explanations as to why they are correlated, one theory is that antiepileptic drugs used to treat bipolar disorder, especially valproate (Depakote), may indirectly promote PCOS.[3,25,35] The incidence of PCOS in women with epilepsy treated with valproate has been shown to be higher than with other antiepileptic drugs.[35]

As for mechanism of action, Himelein and Thatcher noted that research points to the effect that prolonged exposure to valproate has on the ovaries; there is an increased ovarian androgen biosynthesis with sustained exposure to valproate.[3]

Anxiety

Women with PCOS tend to experience more anxiety than women without PCOS.[35-37] In their meta-analysis, Dokras and colleagues found a significantly higher prevalence of anxiety symptoms in women with PCOS (20.4%) compared with controls (3.9%).[35] Women with PCOS may have an increased risk of anxiety symptoms related to low self-esteem, poor body image and weight, fear of future health problems and infertility, and dermatological symptoms.[35]

The relationship between anxiety and BMI in PCOS is not well known. Barry et al found that women with PCOS with lower BMI had slightly lower rates of anxiety.[36] Anxiety could contribute to emotional eating and bingeing.[10]

According to the DSM-5, the diagnostic criteria for generalized anxiety disorder include at least three of the following six symptoms (with at least some symptoms present on most days for the past six months):

- Restlessness or feeling keyed up or on edge
- Being easily fatigued
- Difficulty concentrating or mind going blank
- Irritability
- Muscle tension
- Sleep disturbances

Anxiety occurs in many forms, such as panic attacks, agoraphobia, posttraumatic stress disorder, acute stress disorder, social anxiety, and generalized anxiety. Dokras et al indicated that anxiety symptoms develop over a period of time and may not be identified until they cause problems with functioning.[36] Sleep disturbances are common in PCOS and related to anxiety. Improving sleep disturbances can alleviate fatigue and depressed mood.[15]

Women with PCOS should be routinely screened for anxiety by a mental health professional.

TREATMENT FOR PSYCHOLOGICAL ISSUES

Psychological issues can be managed in many ways, ranging from psychotherapy and psychopharmacology to complementary and alternative medicine (CAM). Psychotherapy is a formal, interpersonal, unilateral, systematic, time-limited relationship that focuses on an individual's problematic behaviors, thoughts, or feelings with efforts to help the individual change.

While there are numerous schools of thought or theories behind psychotherapy methods, strategies, and techniques, there are many that have empirical support in treating particular psychological disorders.

In addition to talk therapies, psychopharmacology has been successful in creating change in psychological conditions as well. Various medications have been found to be effective for treating both anxiety and mood.

Many women diagnosed with PCOS may seek alternative treatments, such as homeopathy or herbal supplements, to assist them with their feelings and emotions. More information on these topics can be found in Chapter 3.

Psychotherapy

As mentioned previously, psychotherapy comes in a variety of forms. Within the past two decades, the American Psychiatric Association has worked on gathering information related to psychotherapy efficacy.[23] Through this process, a considerable amount of information has been discovered about which psychotherapy treatments are effective for particular disorders and which psychotherapy treatments show promise. In addition, this movement in developing empirically supported treatments has motivated clinicians and researchers to conduct similar experiments in a continued effort to develop effective psychotherapies.

For the treatment of depression, behavioral treatment, CBT, and interpersonal psychotherapy have found empirical support. For anxiety and stress-related disorders, cognitive therapy for panic, applied relaxation for panic, exposure treatment for agoraphobia, CBT for generalized anxiety disorder, exposure for social phobia, stress inoculation training for coping with stressors, exposure and response prevention for obsessive compulsive disorder, exposure/ guided imagery for specific phobia, and systematic desensitization for specific phobia have found empirical research. CBT and interpersonal therapy for bulimia nervosa have been found to be efficacious.

There are additional therapies that have showed promise in the treatment literature. Marsha Linehan originally developed dialectical behavior therapy (DBT) for the treatment of parasuicidal and suicidal women. Since its inception, it has undergone rigorous studies and has found an application with bulimia and BED.[39]

DBT may be effective for women with PCOS, as it would teach them how to be mindful of various internal and external stimuli in a nonjudgmental manner while being able to engage in effective behaviors. Patients are taught how to "chain" troublesome situations by identifying negative behaviors interfering with their quality of life as well as those that are life threatening. Women with PCOS may find this aspect most helpful. After identifying negative behaviors, they would learn how to implement emotion regulation, interpersonal effectiveness, and distress tolerance strategies to create a life worth living.

Mindfulness-based stress reduction (MBSR) uses the concept of mindfulness meditation as a skill to reduce both psychological and physical stress. Developed by Jon Kabat-Zinn in 1979, this eight-week program has demonstrated remarkable changes in job-related stress, people with physical conditions such as heart disease and high blood pressure, as well as anxiety substance abuse. MBSR may be helpful for women with PCOS, as it would teach them how to be mindful of their bodies, eating patterns, and state of being.

Support groups for women diagnosed with PCOS can be helpful as well. This type of group would ideally have a mental health professional as the group leader, assisting patients in normalizing each other's experiences and validating emotional responses. In this group, women can impart new information about doctors and specialists as well as try out new interpersonal skills to aid them in the world. It can offer to them the opportunity to be part of a social network as well assist them in learning various new coping strategies. This concept of learning new coping strategies to deal with the PCOS diagnosis, life-changing behaviors and medications, as well as judgments that these patients may have is important.

Psychopharmacology

With the advent of neuroscience and psychiatry, knowledge about psychiatric processes has grown exponentially. Additionally, the field of psychopharmacology has expanded greatly over the past 20 years. Medications for various psychological conditions are plentiful. For those prescribing medications, the process of observing symptoms, assessing the course of illness, and evaluating the risk-to-benefit ratio is critical.[40]

Medications for mood disorders come in different classes, including tricyclics and heterocyclics such as amitriptyline (Elavil) or buproprion (Wellbutrin), selective serotonin reuptake inhibitors (or SSRIs) such as fluoxetine (Prozac) and sertraline (Zoloft), and monoamine oxidase inhibitors (or MAOIs) such as tranylcypromine (Parnate) and phenelzine (Nardil). Each of these medications has a different mechanism of action and different adverse reactions.

Mood stabilizers are primarily used for bipolar disorders, the most common being lithium carbonate and lamotrigine (Lamictal). As mentioned earlier, some of these mood stabilizers have been thought to cause PCOS symptoms. In any case, most have potential side effects that may influence insulin resistance, weight gain, and weight loss.

Medications for anxiety are called antianxiety and sedative-hypnotic agents.[40] Introduced nearly 30 years ago, benzodiazepines were identified as having fewer drawbacks than other medications and were considered safer in combination with other agents. Today, these medications are still the most widely prescribed in terms of reducing anxiety. SSRIs such as sertraline, paroxetine (Paxil), and escitalopram (Lexapro) are also prescribed for anxiety.

Consulting with a knowledgeable psychiatrist is advised if you believe a patient may need medication to address her moods, thoughts, or emotions.

Complementary and Alternative Medicine

CAM refers to the different mind/body strategies that are not generally practiced in western medicine. It is an umbrella term that covers a variety of treatment strategies, such as Theta Healing, acupuncture, herbal and dietary supplements, homeopathy, mindfulness, and Reiki. These treatments can be useful for dietitians because they are often readily available, easy to implement, and can be learned fairly quickly. CAM treatments may improve the endocrine, cardiometabolic, and reproductive aspects of PCOS as well as enhance psychological health and well-being.[41]

Mindfulness has not yet been studied in the PCOS population. Mindfulness, and specifically MBSR programs, have been shown to reduce psychological distress[42] and improve some medical conditions.[41]

More information on CAM treatments can be found in Chapter 3.

In summary, women with PCOS suffer from more emotional stress than women without the syndrome. Anxiety, depression, eating disorders, and bipolar disorder are more prevalent in the PCOS population. Many of these conditions are related to embarrassing dermatological symptoms, weight gain, health problems, and infertility.

Dietitians should be familiar with these mental health disorders so they can recognize them in their patients. If a mental health issue is suspected, dietitians and other health care providers should refer patients to the appropriate mental health expert. Early detection and treatment are crucial.

CHAPTER SUMMARY

- Infertility, weight, and the dermatological symptoms women with PCOS experience have a direct effect on body image and self-esteem.
- Women with PCOS have a greater prevalence of anxiety, depression, and bipolar disorder than other women.
- Eating disorders are common among the PCOS population.
- The risk of suicide is high among women with PCOS.
- There are different treatment strategies available for women with PCOS, including prescription medications, psychotherapy, and complementary and alternative medicines.
- Patients suspected of mental health issues should be referred to a mental health professional for assessment and treatment.

REFERENCES

1. Rassi A, Veras AB, dos Reis M, et al. Prevalence of psychiatric disorders in patients with polycystic ovary syndrome. Compr. Psychiatry. 2010;51(6):599-602.

2. Brady C, Mousa SS, Mousa SA. Polycystic ovary syndrome and its impact on women's quality of life: More than just an endocrine disorder. Drug Healthc Patient Saf. 2009;1:9-15.

3. Himelein MJ, Thatcher SS. Depression and body image among women with polycystic ovary syndrome. J. Health Psychol. 2006;11(4):613-625.

4. Himelein MJ, Thatcher SS. Polycystic ovary syndrome and mental health: A review. Obstet. Gynecol. Surv. 2006;61(11):723-732.

5. Cipkala-Gaffin J, Talbott EO, Song MK, Bromberger J, Wilson J. Associations between psychologic symptoms and life satisfaction in women with polycystic ovary syndrome. J Womens Health. 2012;21(2):179-187.

6. Jones GL, Hall JM, Balen AH, Ledger WL. Health-related quality of life measurement in women with polycystic ovary syndrome: a systematic review. Hum. Reprod. Update. 2008;14(1):15-25.

7. Li Y, Li Y, Yu Ng EH, et al. Polycystic ovary syndrome is associated with negatively variable impacts on domains of health-related quality of life: evidence from a meta-analysis. Fertil. Steril. 2011;96(2):452-458.

8. Raison CL, Capuron L, Miller AH. Cytokines sing the blues: inflammation and the pathogenesis of depression. Trends Immunol. 2006;27(1):24-31.

9. Zorrilla EP, Luborsky L, McKay JR, et al. The relationship of depression and stressors to immunological assays: a meta-analytic review. Brain. Behav. Immun. 2001;15(3):199-226.

10. Kocelak P, Chudek J, Naworska B, et al. Psychological disturbances and quality of life in obese and infertile women and men. Int. J. Endocrinol. 2012;2012:236217.

11. Rutledge T, Linden W. To eat or not to eat: affective and physiological mechanisms in the stress-eating relationship. J. Behav. Med. 1998;21(3):221-240.

12. Moore CJ, Cunningham SA. Social position, psychological stress, and obesity: a systematic review. J Acad Nutr Diet. 2012;112(4):518-526.

13. Epel E, Lapidus R, McEwen B, Brownell K. Stress may add bite to appetite in women: a laboratory study of stress-induced cortisol and eating behavior. Psychoneuroendocrinology. 2001;26(1):37-49.

14. Benson S, Arck PC, Tan S, et al. Disturbed stress responses in women with polycystic ovary syndrome. Psychoneuroendocrinology. 2009;34(5):727-735.

15. Farrell K, Antoni MH. Insulin resistance, obesity, inflammation, and

depression in polycystic ovary syndrome: biobehavioral mechanisms and interventions. Fertil. Steril. 2010;94(5):1565-1574.

16. Drapeau V, Therrien F, Richard D, Tremblay A. Is visceral obesity a physiological adaptation to stress? Panminerva Med. 2003;45(3):189-195.

17. Lipton MG, Sherr L, Elford J, Rustin MHA, Clayton WJ. Women living with facial hair: the psychological and behavioral burden. J. Psychosom. Res. 2006;61(2):161-168.

18. Connolly KJ, Edelmann RJ, Cooke ID, Robson J. The impact of infertility on psychological functioning. J. Psychosom. Res. 1992;36(5):459-468.

19. Trent ME, Rich M, Austin SB, Gordon CM. Fertility concerns and sexual behavior in adolescent girls with polycystic ovary syndrome: implications for quality of life. J. Pediatr. Adolesc. Gynecol. 2003;16(1):33-37.

20. Elsenbruch S, Hahn S, Kowalsky D, et al. Quality of life, psychosocial well-being, and sexual satisfaction in women with polycystic ovary syndrome. J. Clin. Endocrinol. Metab. 2003;88(12):5801-5807.

21. Conaglen HM, Conaglen JV. Sexual medicine: Why stop a good thing? Discontinuing PDE5 inhibitors. Nat Rev Urol. 2012;9(9):483-485.

22. Homburg R. The management of infertility associated with polycystic ovary syndrome. Reprod. Biol. Endocrinol. 2003;1:109.

23. Chambless DL, Baker, M. J., Baucom, D. H., Beutler, L. E., Calhoun, K. S., Crits-Christoph, P., Daiuto, A., DeRubeis, R., Detweiler, J., Haaga, D. A. F., Bennett Johnson, S., McCurry, S., Mueser, K. T., Pope, K. S., Sanderson, W. C., Shoham, V., Stickle, T., Williams, D. A., & Woody, S. R. Update on empirically validated therapies, II. The Clinical Psychologist. 1998;51(1):3-16.

24. Woody SR W, McLean C. . Empirically supported treatments: 10 years later. The Clinical Psychologist. 2005;58(4):5-11.

25. Rasgon NL, Rao RC, Hwang S, et al. Depression in women with polycystic ovary syndrome: clinical and biochemical correlates. J. Affect. Disord. 2003;74(3):299-304.

26. Association AP. DSM. 5th ed. Washington D.C.: American Psychological Association 2013.

27. Spitzer RL, Devlin, M., Walsh, B. T., Hasin, D., Wing, R., Marcus, M., Stunkard, A., Wadden, T., Yanovski, S., Agras, S., Mitchell, J. and Nonas, C. Binge eating disorder: A multisite field trial of the diagnostic criteria. Int. J. Eat. Disord. 1992;11:191–203.

28. Kerchner A, Lester W, Stuart SP, Dokras A. Risk of depression and other mental health disorders in women with polycystic ovary syndrome: a longitudinal study. Fertil. Steril. 2009;91(1):207-212.

29. Mansson M, Holte J, Landin-Wilhelmsen K, Dahlgren E, Johansson A, Landen M. Women with polycystic ovary syndrome are often depressed or anxious--a case control study. Psychoneuroendocrinology. 2008;33(8):1132-1138.

30. Brown AJ. Depression and insulin resistance: applications to polycystic ovary syndrome. Clin. Obstet. Gynecol. 2004;47(3):592-596.

31. Okamura F, Tashiro A, Utumi A, et al. Insulin resistance in patients with depression and its changes during the clinical course of depression: minimal model analysis. Metabolism. 2000;49(10):1255-1260.

32. Amsterdam JD, Shults J, Rutherford N, Schwartz S. Safety and efficacy of s-citalopram in patients with co-morbid major depression and diabetes mellitus. Neuropsychobiology. 2006;54(4):208-214.

33. Keegan A, Liao L-M, Boyle M. 'Hirsutism': a psychological analysis. J. Health Psychol. 2003;8(3):327-345.

34. Weiner CL, Primeau M, Ehrmann DA. Androgens and mood dysfunction in women: comparison of women with polycystic ovarian syndrome to healthy controls. Psychosom. Med. 2004;66(3):356-362.

35. Hu X, Wang J, Dong W, Fang Q, Hu L, Liu C. A meta-analysis of polycystic ovary syndrome in women taking valproate for epilepsy. Epilepsy Res. 2011;97(1-2):73-82.

36. Dokras A, Clifton S, Futterweit W, Wild R. Increased prevalence of anxiety symptoms in women with polycystic ovary syndrome: systematic review and meta-analysis. Fertil. Steril. 2012;97(1):225-230.

37. Barry JA, Kuczmierczyk AR, Hardiman PJ. Anxiety and depression in polycystic ovary syndrome: a systematic review and meta-analysis. Hum. Reprod. 2011;26(9):2442-2451.

38. Veltman-Verhulst SM, Boivin J, Eijkemans MJ, Fauser BJ. Emotional distress is a common risk in women with polycystic ovary syndrome: a systematic review and meta-analysis of 28 studies. Hum. Reprod. Update. 2012;18(6):638-651.

39. Telch CF, Agras WS, Linehan MM. Dialectical behavior therapy for binge eating disorder. J. Consult. Clin. Psychol. 2001;69(6):1061-1065.

40. Janiack PG DJ, Preshkorn SH, Ayd FJ. Principles and practice of psychopharacotherapy. Philadelphia, PA: Lippincott Williams & Wilkins; 1997.

41. Raja-Khan N, Stener-Victorin E, Wu X, Legro RS. The physiological basis of complementary and alternative medicines for polycystic ovary syndrome. Am. J. Physiol. Endocrinol. Metab. 2011;301(1):E1-E10.

42. Ludwig DS, Kabat-Zinn J. Mindfulness in medicine. JAMA. 2008;300(11):1350-1352.

Chapter 8

PCOS AND EATING DISORDERS

The first time I heard about PCOS was in 1999 while working for an eating disorder treatment facility. A patient named Sarah, 27, tearfully explained to me the symptoms she was experiencing: severe acne and hair growth on her face, absent periods, thinning hair, weight increases of roughly 2 lbs per month for the last year. She hated her body and felt it was out of control.

She had been diagnosed with PCOS three weeks earlier, and her doctor recommended that she try the Atkins low-carbohydrate diet to manage her insulin and help her lose weight. Through the tears, Sarah admitted that she had tried to follow the diet but that she kept bingeing on carbohydrates and felt so guilty afterward that she purged to get rid of them. Sarah also had a long history of bulimia nervosa.

MENSTRUAL DISTURBANCES

It is widely accepted that women with eating disorders or a combination of several symptoms of eating disorders, commonly referred to as eating disorder not otherwise specified (EDNOS), or other specified feeding or eating disorder (OSFED), experience menstrual disturbances.[1-4] Much like women with PCOS, these menstrual disturbances include anovulation and oligomenorrhea.[5]

Resch et al examined the hormonal dysfunction associated with improper eating habits among 14 subjects with bulimia nervosa and 22 subjects with EDNOS.[5] They found decreased levels of FSH and LH among both groups, while the EDNOS group had the lowest levels of the two hormones and higher amounts of testosterone than controls.

The researchers suggested that one reason many women with bulimia and EDNOS may have menstrual disturbances is related to low levels of LH, which is a sensitive variant affected by dramatic changes in eating habits.[5] Thus, crash dieting or restricting, which are common bulimic and compulsive eating behaviors, may affect levels of LH. This can result in an insufficient luteal phase, producing the oligomenorrhea or anovulation seen in PCOS.

THE EMOTIONAL TOLL

Like Sarah, the symptoms many women with PCOS endure can have a direct effect on their body image and self-esteem, and may lead to the development of distorted eating habits or eating disorders, linking the two conditions.[6] There seems to be a genetic component to the development of PCOS, with studies indicating that some girls are even born with polycystic-appearing ovaries.[7]

Most symptoms, however, do not appear until the onset of puberty—another factor in common with eating disorders. For example, at a time when a young woman's self-esteem is vulnerable, she may start to experience acne and excessive hair growth on her face and other parts of her body along with weight gain in her midsection, setting her apart from her peers. Not knowing that she has PCOS or why she is experiencing such phenomena, she may begin to blame herself and hate her body. Struggling with these issues at such a vulnerable time can lead many young women to deal with their emotional distress through unhealthful dieting practices such as laxatives, diuretics, diet pills, fasting, excessive exercise, and vomiting. These negative behaviors can set the stage for a lifetime of eating issues and body hatred.

The relationship between monozygotic and dizygotic twins with PCOS and bulimia was investigated by using the BITE questionnaire (Bulimia Investigation Test, Edinburgh), a self-rating scale used to diagnose bulimia that includes 30 questions about dieting and binge behaviors, such as "Does your pattern of eating severely disrupt your life?" "Do you ever experience overpowering urges to eat and eat?" and "Do you ever fast for a whole day?"[8]

Results showed 76% of twins with PCOS had elevated scores on the BITE questionnaire, suggesting that a relationship does exist between bulimia and PCOS. Other studies conducted using the BITE questionnaire support a relationship between PCOS and binge eating, with one-third of women with PCOS in one study demonstrating binge-eating behavior.[9]

The development of binge eating among women with PCOS is all too common. Many are frustrated with their diagnosis. They feel immense pressure because they desperately want to lose weight, conceive a child, and improve their symptoms overall. They believe the only way to do this is by dieting.

Often times they will restrict carbohydrates to lose weight or sometimes they eat limited amounts of food. This, combined with carbohydrate cravings and hypoglycemia, results in bingeing and feeling even worse about themselves. After consuming large amounts of food and feeling the guilt associated with a binge, they tend to want to restrict their intake, purge, or engage in other unhealthy behaviors to get rid of the overwhelming feelings. This, in turn, can set them up for another binge episode. Thus a vicious cycle ensues.

On the other hand, many women with PCOS have a long history of yo-yo dieting. Even before knowing they had PCOS, they struggled with their weight, either trying to prevent the number on the scale from creeping up or trying to make it go down, only to lose weight and gain it back. The result of being on so many different diets, each time looking for a quick fix, is that they learn to view foods as good or bad. Therefore, they feel guilty if they eat certain bad foods and, in turn, feel bad about themselves. They also learn not to trust their bodies as to when they need food, how much food they need, and whether they need it.

Women with PCOS may be more prone to mood swings and depression than someone without PCOS. As discussed in Chapter 7, mental health problems are common among individuals with eating disorders. Also, having elevated testosterone may make women with PCOS more aggressive, angry, anxious, and depressed. Many women with PCOS, however, may also have mood disturbances from dealing with the symptoms associated with their diagnosis.[10] Patients may benefit from consulting with a psychiatrist to assess the use of medications in addition to regularly working with a therapist.

THE INSULIN EFFECT

It is understandable that women with PCOS may become more susceptible to developing an eating disorder and suffer from body image disturbances, but can women with eating disorders develop PCOS?

It has been proposed that insulin may have an appetite-stimulating effect and can perpetuate binge behavior.[1] For example, during an eating binge, when large quantities of food are consumed over a relatively short amount of time, there is a surge of excess insulin, much more than experienced during a normal meal. Constant bingeing could, therefore, result in a chronic state of elevated insulin. Hyperinsulinemia stimulates the ovaries to produce more androgens,[1] which are also known to have appetite-stimulating effects.[11] As a result, women with PCOS who engage in binge eating will further increase insulin levels and worsen their PCOS symptoms.

Rapheal et al investigated whether women with bulimia are insulin resistant and examined the relationship between insulin and androgen levels, ovarian morphology, and the severity of bulimic behavior.[1] Although they did not find that women with bulimia had insulin resistance, they did find that they were chronically hyperinsulinemic, with 10 of their 12 normal-weight subjects having polycystic ovaries.[5] This led the researchers to speculate that hyperinsulinemia may be one reason a connection exists between bulimia and PCOS. The bulimic pattern of bingeing followed by starvation and/or vomiting perpetuates the insulin response and leads to the development of polycystic ovaries.[1] It may also suggest why some women who are overweight or obese without a family history develop PCOS through overfeeding.

There is some encouraging news: it appears that when women with PCOS and bulimia return to normalized eating patterns with treatment involving CBT, it can result in improved ovarian morphology.[3] Chronic bingeing can worsen the appearance of polycystic ovaries, but ovarian morphology does seem to resolve when binging ceases and normal eating patterns are established.

IMPAIRED APPETITE REGULATION

Research has suggested that women with PCOS have impaired appetite regulation.[11-15] Impaired secretion of the hormone CCK has been demonstrated in PCOS, resulting in a reduced feeling of satiety.[11,12] CCK is released from the small intestine in response to the presence of food and plays an important role in regulating appetite. It has been shown that women with bulimia nervosa have impaired CCK secretion,[12] which could also explain why women with PCOS, bulimia, or EDNOS tend to crave sweets, binge eat, or be overweight: because of their impaired ability to feel full.

It is not known why women with PCOS have impaired CCK secretion following meals, but it has been suggested that like individuals with bulimia and diabetes, women with PCOS may have delayed gastric emptying.[11]

Impaired levels ghrelin[13,14] have also been documented in PCOS, further suggesting that women with PCOS have appetite abnormalities.[13,14] Fasting levels of ghrelin have been found to be impaired in lean and obese women with PCOS compared with weight-matched women without PCOS.[13] In one study, women with PCOS who were overweight were less satiated and hungrier after test meals than those without PCOS.[13]

Leptin, a protein hormone involved in energy balance secreted to signal satiety, is also compromised in women with PCOS.[15] A positive correlation exists between leptin and BMI and between leptin and testosterone in women with PCOS.[15] Decreased leptin function may stimulate eating in women with PCOS, resulting in increased food intake and difficulty managing weight.[16] In addition, having impaired levels of CCK and ghrelin could possibly explain women with PCOS have trouble losing weight: appetite signals are compromised, making them hungrier and wanting to eat more.

Interestingly, a relationship has been documented among leptin, eating disorders, and PCOS.[17] Leptin concentrations in women with anorexia nervosa have been found to be lower than those of normal-weight controls.[18] Leptin may even be implicated in the pathophysiology of PCOS because it is also involved in reproductive function.[19]

SCREENING FOR DISTORTED EATING

Because women with PCOS may be more prone to binge eating, it is imperative that dietitians screen these patients before recommending a dietary plan or changes in eating behavior. Effective questions to ask during the initial assessment include the following:

- "Tell me how you feel about your weight."
- "Describe your control of food."
- "Tell me about your feelings of hunger and fullness."
- "How do you feel about eating foods containing carbohydrates?"
- "Tell me about any methods you use to control your weight."
- "How do you feel when you eat with other people?"
- "How do you feel when you eat while doing something else at the same time (e.g., watching TV or using the computer)?"

If distorted eating is suspected, initial focus should be on normalizing eating patterns to control insulin levels and prevent bingeing and weight gain. Even without focusing on weight loss, ovarian morphology and insulin levels may improve by restoring normal eating patterns.[3] Many of the physicians I work with prefer to monitor clients' insulin and HbA1c levels, in addition to liver function tests, approximately every three months. This can be a valuable for reflecting changes in a client's eating pattern and a motivating tool to show a client that although she may not have lost weight, the positive changes she has made in her eating have resulted in health improvements.

Clients need to be educated on the importance of structuring regular meals and snacks throughout the day to stabilize blood sugar levels and prevent cravings and hypoglycemic episodes. This may include eating every three to five hours and adding protein and fat to meals and snacks.[20]

Some clients may benefit from planning their meals and snacks ahead of time; this can reduce anxiety and give the client a better sense of comfort, knowing that more food is available later.

In addition, I have noticed that many of my clients with PCOS who take insulin-lowering medications such as metformin report less carbohydrate cravings and reduced interest in food overall.

Because of their struggles maintaining weight through dieting, many women with PCOS may have lost their internal ability to regulate food intake. For example, they may not be able to effectively distinguish when they are hungry. This could result in them eating when they don't need to or waiting long periods to eat. If they do use food to cope with emotions, perhaps they are unable to distinguish when they are physically satisfied with food, leading them to eat more than they need to. Therefore, establishing life-long normalized eating patterns should involve education and support with mindful eating.

Food Logs

The use of food logs to rate hunger and satisfaction levels before and after meals can be an effective technique for promoting self-awareness. I encourage my clients to use a scale from 0 to 10, with 0 equating to extreme hunger, 5 being neutral (not hungry or full), and 10 being Thanksgiving-dinner stuffed. They should assess their rating throughout the day, especially before, during, and after meals, to determine when they need to eat and how much.

Chances are that women who have kept food logs in the past either for various diet plans or for their own use have not previously monitored their hunger or satiety levels. Checking hunger and satiety can be difficult and practically impossible at first for women with PCOS who have dieted throughout their life. It is important to let a client know that it may be difficult for her to do this at first, but it is a process that she can practice and experiment with to eventually be able to listen and respond to her internal cues.

Reviewing food logs together can help clients identify whether they are eating when they do not need to, eating for emotional reasons, or eating enough at a meal to feel satisfied. This also provides a great opportunity to explore and challenge a client's attitude toward food and weight.

Conscious Eating Exercises

Conscious eating exercises are another way to reinforce mindful eating. Exercises can be done during nutrition sessions and practiced at home. This means eating food together either as a meal or a snack and helping a client to consciously recognize how food tastes and feels to her. I have even done this using a cracker, raisin, grape, or piece of chocolate.

These exercises can be extremely beneficial for a woman who often eats on the run, while standing, or while in front of her TV or computer screen. Usually, when people eat while they are doing something such as watching TV or driving, they must focus on what is in front of them and therefore do not focus on tasting the food.

After completing the conscious eating exercise, I will discuss with clients how it feels to eat mindfully rather than while distracted. It really is an eye-opening exercise. Clients report experiencing the texture and taste of food as if they ate it for the first time.

I discuss conscious eating exercises with clients during one session and then have them bring food to subsequent planned sessions. (I keep snacks in my office too). I bring my own food and usually eat with my clients. I find this to be a great way to model mindful eating, and it makes the client feel more comfortable than having to eat by herself.

To begin a mindful eating or conscious eating exercise during a nutrition session, I start by having the client set up her food, drink, and utensils on the table. Next I lead her through a relaxation exercise or encourage deep breathing.

I then have the client examine the food that she brought by observing the color, shape, and texture. The next step is for her to pick up part of the food and, if she can, feel its texture. Finally, I instruct the client to place the bite of food (or grape or cracker) in her mouth, noting the feel and texture of that food prior to chewing. She can then start slowly chewing the food and swallowing, again noting any feelings or sensations she experiences.

The client repeats the exercise by eating mindfully with each bite of food. She is encouraged to practice this outside of nutrition sessions by using her food log to rate her degree of hunger and satisfaction level before and after meals. To effectively practice these exercises, eating should be done in a relaxed setting at a table and away from distractions.

Challenging Negative Thoughts

Because of their history with dieting, many women with PCOS may have some negative and false beliefs about food. Some of these beliefs may include that they can't eat foods containing carbohydrates, carbs are bad, they can't eat fruit because it has carbs, and fat is bad.

As dietitians, we need to provide objective and reliable nutrition information and clear up any false beliefs, especially when they directly affect a client's health. For example, educating your client that even though fruit contains carbohydrates, women with PCOS should not avoid it because of the fiber and other beneficial nutrients.

Women with PCOS may fear carbohydrates, believing they must limit their intake of all carbohydrate sources. This is particularly problematic for a woman with a history of an eating disorder or, as discussed earlier, can lead to the development of an eating disorder. It may be in the client's best interest to include some form of a whole grain carbohydrate source at each meal or snack at first to help her break a binge or binge-purge cycle, regulate blood sugar levels, and avoid hypoglycemia.

Additionally, some clients may fear that if they add carbohydrates back into their diet they will lose control and start bingeing on them. It is important for them to know that it is fine to eat carbohydrates again and why they are beneficial. Additionally, these clients should add carbohydrates gradually, starting with those that are "safest" to them.

Coping Skills

Most of all, women struggling with PCOS and an eating disorder need to learn effective ways to deal with their emotions without abusing food. Dietitians can help clients identify possible alternative coping skills and should support clients with instituting them. For example, I have my clients make a list of positive things they can do when they feel like bingeing. This may include activities such as taking a walk, reading, journaling, calling a friend, surfing the Internet, or taking a bath. In addition, working with a psychotherapist may help individuals identify their emotional triggers, and encourage mindfulness and behavior change.

Once normalized eating patterns have been established and clients can safely respond to internal cues of hunger and satiety, further recommendations on diet and exercise may be advised with caution and should focus on continuing to improve overall health rather than weight loss.[21,22]

In summary, there is a high risk of eating disorders among the PCOS population. All women with PCOS should be screened for distorted eating and eating disorders. If suspected, the initial focus should be on normalizing eating patterns to control insulin levels and prevent bingeing and weight gain. Even without focusing on weight loss, ovarian morphology and insulin levels may improve by restoring normal eating patterns. Dietitians can help clients normalize their eating through the use of conscious eating exercises, coping skills, cognitive restructuring techniques, and reality checks.

CHAPTER SUMMARY

- Erratic eating habits, such as periods of restricting followed by bingeing and/or purging, can affect hormones and cause menstrual disturbances.
- Women with PCOS have a higher risk of developing an eating disorder or distorted eating because of the detrimental effects of their symptoms on body image, weight, and mood disturbances.
- Insulin has an appetite-stimulating effect and may make women with PCOS more prone to binge eating, especially when engaging in restrictive eating.
- PCOS women have impaired secretion of CCK, leptin, and ghrelin, thus affecting appetite regulation.
- It is imperative that dietitians screen patients with PCOS for eating disorders before recommending dieting or changes in eating behavior.

REFERENCES

1. Raphael FJ, Rodin DA, Peattie A, et al. Ovarian morphology and insulin sensitivity in women with bulimia nervosa. Clin Endocrinol (Oxf). 1995;43(4):451-455.

2. Michelmore KF, Balen AH, Dunger DB. Polycystic ovaries and eating disorders: are they related? Human Repro. 2001;16(4):765-769.

3. Morgan JF, McCluskey SE, Brunton JN, Hubert Lacey J. Polycystic ovarian morphology and bulimia nervosa: a 9-year follow-up study. Fertil Steril. 2002;77(5):928-931.

4. Naessen S, Carlstrom K, Garoff L, Glant R, Hirschberg AL. Polycystic ovary syndrome in bulimic women--an evaluation based on the new diagnostic criteria. Gynecol Endocrinol. 2006;22(7):388-394.

5. Resch M, Szendei G, Haasz P. Bulimia from a gynecological view: hormonal changes. Journal of obstetrics and gynaecology. J. Institute Obstet Gynaecol. 2004;24(8):907-910.

6. McCluskey S, Evans C, Lacey JH, Pearce JM, Jacobs H. Polycystic ovary syndrome and bulimia. Fertil Steril. 1991;55(2):287-291.

7. Bridges NA, Cooke A, Healy MJ, Hindmarsh PC, Brook CG. Standards for ovarian volume in childhood and puberty. Fertili Steril. 1993;60(3):456-460.

8. Jahanfar S, Eden JA, Nguyent TV. Bulimia nervosa and polycystic ovary syndrome. Gynecol Endocrinol. 1995;9(2):113-117.

9. McCluskey SE, Lacey JH, Pearce JM. Binge-eating and polycystic ovaries. Lancet. 1992;340(8821):723.

10. Weiner CL, Primeau M, Ehrmann DA. Androgens and mood dysfunction in women: comparison of women with polycystic ovarian syndrome to healthy controls. Psychosomatic medicine. 2004;66(3):356-362.

11. Hirschberg AL, Naessen S, Stridsberg M, Bystrom B, Holtet J. Impaired cholecystokinin secretion and disturbed appetite regulation in women with polycystic ovary syndrome. Gynecol Endocrinol. 2004;19(2):79-87.

12. Geracioti TD, Jr., Liddle RA. Impaired cholecystokinin secretion in bulimia nervosa. NEJM. 1988;319(11):683-688.

13. Moran LJ, Noakes M, Clifton PM, et al. Ghrelin and measures of satiety are altered in polycystic ovary syndrome but not differentially affected by diet composition. J Clin Endocrinol Metab. 2004;89(7):3337-3344.

14. Moran LJ, Noakes M, Clifton PM, et al. Postprandial ghrelin, cholecystokinin, peptide YY, and appetite before and after weight loss in

overweight women with and without polycystic ovary syndrome. Amer J
Clin Nutr. 2007;86(6):1603-1610.

15. Baranowska B, Radzikowska M, Wasilewska-Dziubinska E, Kaplinski
A, Roguski K, Plonowski A. Neuropeptide Y, leptin, galanin and
insulin in women with polycystic ovary syndrome. Gynecol Endocrinol.
1999;13(5):344-351.

16. Jahanfar S, Maleki H, Mosavi AR. Subclinical eating disorder, polycystic
ovary syndrome- is there any connection between these two conditions
through leptin- a twin study. Medical J Malaysia. 2005;60(4):441-446.

17. Jaafar SH, Jahanfar S, Angolkar M, Ho JJ. Effect of restricted pacifier use
in breastfeeding term infants for increasing duration of breastfeeding.
Cochrane Database Syst Rev. 2012;7.

18. Amsterdam JD, Shults J, Rutherford N, Schwartz S. Safety and efficacy of
s-citalopram in patients with co-morbid major depression and diabetes
mellitus. Neuropsychobiology. 2006;54(4):208-214.

19. Hausman GJ, Barb CR, Lents CA. Leptin and reproductive function.
Biochimie. 2012;94(10):2075-2081.

20. Marsh K, Brand-Miller J. The optimal diet for women with polycystic ovary
syndrome? BJN. 2005;94(2):154-165.

21. Morgan J. Bulimic eating patterns should be stabilized in polycystic ovary
syndrome. BMJ. 1999;318:328.

22. Moran L, Norman RJ. Understanding and managing disturbances in
insulin metabolism and body weight in women with polycystic ovary
syndrome. Best Pract Res Clin Obstet Gynaecol. 2004;18(5):719-736.

Chapter 9
_____

CASE STUDIES

By Angela Grassi, MS, RD, LDN;
Lynn Monahan Couch, DCN, MPH, RD, LDN;
Judy Simon, MS, RD, CDE, CHES

This chapter discusses three separate case studies in which MNT was provided to patients with PCOS.

In the first case study, a young woman named Gita seeks help for weight loss and a diet to improve fertility, only to become pregnant during the course of treatment.

The second case study involves an adolescent, Carrie, with a history of binge eating who begins nutrition counseling for weight loss. Nutrition strategies involve helping her normalize her eating while improving her health.

Finally, the third case involves Melissa, a woman who is obese and presents with many adverse health conditions associated with PCOS. MNT interventions focused on helping her change her eating and lifestyle behaviors to reduce her risk of disease.

CASE 1

Gita was a 27-year-old East Indian female with PCOS who was referred to a dietitian by her reproductive endocrinologist for weight loss and fertility. Gita had gained 10 lbs over the past year since moving to Washington state with her husband and parents. She had been trying to conceive since her miscarriage one year before. Her last pregnancy was conceived without fertility assistance.

For religious reasons, Gita followed a vegetarian diet and avoided eggs; she disliked milk. Most dinners were eaten with her husband

and parents, who lived in her apartment complex, and consisted of traditional home-prepared Indian foods. Lunch consisted of leftovers from dinner or a sandwich and chips if out with her mother. Gita reported strong cravings for carbohydrates and juice.

Gita did not work outside the home and, other than house chores, was sedentary. Her physician recommended that she increase her physical activity, and she started using the elliptical in her apartment complex two days per week for 20 minutes.

She experienced irregular menstrual cycles. She wanted to lose weight and improve her ovulation before undergoing invasive and costly fertility treatments.

Nutritional Assessment Data

1. Anthropometric Measurements
Height: 5'3"
Weight: 162 lbs
Usual weight: 132 lbs
BMI: 28.7
Waist: 39.6"
Hips: 42.8"

2. Biochemical Data:

Parameter	Value	Normal Values (may vary by age, sex, and laboratory)
Total Testosterone	82	2-45 ng/dL
25(OH)D	11	30-100 nd/mL
HbA1C	5.5	4.0 - 6.0%
Glucose (fasting)	89	65-99 mg/dL
2 Hour Glucose	91	<120 mg/dl
Total Cholesterol	188	<200 mg/dL
LDL Cholesterol	100	<130 mg/dL
Triglycerides	210	<150 mg/dL

3. Nutrition-Focused Physical Findings

Patient has visible excess abdominal fat and excessive facial hair.

4. Client History

Gita is a 27-year-old married woman who wanted to lose weight and improve her fertility. She had suffered a miscarriage one year prior. She experienced a 10-lb weight gain this year. She is inactive.

5. Food/Nutrition-Related History

• Usual Diet

Breakfast (8 am)	2 pieces roti flatbread, 8 oz tea with 2 tsp sugar
Lunch (12 pm)	Vegetable curry, 2 cups basmati rice, 8 oz orange juice or 12-in cheese sub with mayo, lettuce, and tomato, small bag of chips, 8 oz juice
Snack (3 pm)	1 granola bar, 1 piece of fruit, 8 oz tea with 2 tsp sugar
Dinner (6 pm)	Vegetable curry, 2 cups basmati rice, 16 oz orange juice, piece of fruit

• Medications: none
• Supplements: prenatal vitamin and 50,000 IU of vitamin D per week (orally) for eight weeks

6. Nutrition Diagnosis

PES1: Excessive carbohydrate intake (NI-53.2) related to knowledge deficit as evidenced by diet history and BMI.

PES2: Physical inactivity (NB-2.1) related to knowledge deficit as evidenced by current physical activity level.

PES3: Inadequate intake of omega-3 fatty acids (NI-54.1) related to hypertriglyceridemia as evidenced by serum triglyceride level.

Nutrition Intervention

The dietitian discussed optimizing nutrition intake and fitness to benefit weight loss, fertility, and PCOS symptoms. The dietitian used comprehensive nutrition education (E-2.0), leading to increased knowledge of carbohydrate counting using Indian educational materials that included her native foods. The dietitian also discussed how carbohydrates impact insulin and glucose levels, and the benefits of adding fiber-rich foods and protein to meals for increased satiety. Food models were used to show appropriate carbohydrate portions.

Gita was encouraged to engage in physical activity for 45 minutes daily four days per week to achieve weight loss and improved fertility. Fish oil supplementation was recommended to reduce triglyceride levels and aid in fertility. Myo-inositol (MYO) was also recommended for improving egg quality and ovulation. Gita agreed to keep food records.

Overall goals for Gita included the following:

- Achieve at least 5% weight loss, which will improve fertility. Monitor weight and waist circumference.
- Reduce carbohydrate consumption at meals to 30 to 45 g. Eliminate juice and sugar from tea. Eat fiber-rich foods and protein with meals. Review food records.
- Increase physical activity up to 45 minutes four days per week.
- Take 2 g of fish oil supplements, 2 g of MYO, a prenatal vitamin, and a vitamin D supplement as prescribed. Review triglyceride and 25(OH)D levels in four months.

Monitoring and Evaluation

Gita kept food records that she e-mailed to the dietitian each week. She reduced her portions of rice by one-half, and eliminated juice and sugar from her tea. She added protein (milk or yogurt) to her meals and complied with daily supplement recommendations. She exercised three days a week for 45 minutes.

She was followed monthly. After four months, lab results showed her triglyceride and vitamin D levels were within normal levels. She lost 12 lbs (8% of her body weight) and 2 inches from her waist. Her menstrual cycle regulated, and she conceived with timed intercourse without fertility assistance.

Gita met with the dietitian during her pregnancy for nutrition counseling. She delivered a healthy, full-term boy. She gained 20 lbs during her pregnancy and did not develop GDM.

CASE 2

Carrie was a 16-year-old with PCOS who received nutrition counseling for weight loss. Since age 8, Carrie struggled with her weight. She followed numerous commercial diet plans with little success. Last summer, Carrie went to a weight loss camp for two months and lost 9 lbs, which she eventually regained. Carrie was inactive. She had a boyfriend but few close friends. She liked to sing and enjoyed music.

Her parents were concerned about Carrie's increasing weight. They would find junk food hidden in her room and candy wrappers in her backpack. Both parents were slender and health conscious. They did not buy junk food and followed a low-carbohydrate diet. However, Carrie was adopted and had a body type different from her parents. Carrie was angry with her parents for trying to manage her food intake. She met with a therapist monthly to discuss her anger and relationship with her parents.

When probed about disordered eating behaviors, Carrie admitted to bingeing on sweets once or twice a week. She also had a history of self-induced vomiting that started when she was in eighth grade. The last time she purged was six months ago. She denied any urges to binge again. She also denied ever using laxatives, diuretics, or diet pills.

Medically speaking, Carrie had irregular periods. She saw a gynecologist recently who prescribed OCPs to regulate her menstrual cycle. Carrie reported feeling very tired and experienced hypoglycemia several times per day. She had strong cravings for carbohydrate foods, saying "I just have to have them." She also had difficulty recognizing when she was full.

Nutritional Assessment Data
1. Anthropometric Measurements
Height: 5'4"
Weight: 225 lbs.
BMI: 38.6
Waist: 44.5"
Hips: 47"

2. Biochemical Data:

Parameter	Value	Normal Values (may vary by age, sex, and laboratory)
Total Testosterone	72	2-45 ng/dL
Glucose (fasting)	92	65-99 mg/dL
HbA1C	5.7	4.0 - 6.0%
25(OH)D	22	30-100 nd/mL
Total Cholesterol	162	<200 mg/dL
HDL Cholesterol	45	>46 mg/dL
LDL Cholesterol	105	<130 mg/dL
Triglycerides	185	<150 mg/dl

3. Nutrition-Focused Physical Findings

Patient has visible excess abdominal fat and acne.

4. Client History

Patient is a 16-year-old high school student and an only child. She has dieted since age 8 and has a history of vomiting. She currently binges one to two times weekly in the afternoon.

5. Food/Nutrition-Related History
  • Usual Diet

Breakfast (6:50 am)	16 oz chocolate milk and granola bar
Lunch (12:45 pm)	Roast beef sandwich (3 oz) on white bread, French fries with French salad dressing, candy bar, 16 oz water
Snack (3 pm)	Salsa and chips, candy bar (bought at vending machine), 12 oz water
Dinner (6:30 pm)	½ cup butternut squash, ½ cup low-calorie applesauce, 6 oz grilled chicken, 12 oz seltzer water

Dietary assessment showed Carrie consumed high amounts of saturated fat, sodium, and refined carbohydrates. Her fruit and vegetable intake was limited, and her calcium and omega-3 fat intake was below required amounts. There were long periods between breakfast and lunch; her afternoon snack consisted of refined carbohydrates.

- Medications: OCPs
- Supplements: none

Nutrition Diagnosis

PES1: Distorted eating behavior (NB-1.5) related to excessive energy intake of carbohydrate-dense foods as evidenced by binge eating one to two times weekly.

PES2: Excessive carbohydrate intake (NI-53.2) related to knowledge deficit as evidenced by diet history and BMI of 38.6.

PES3: Inadequate intake of omega-3 fatty acids (NI-54.1) related to hypertriglyceridemia as evidenced by serum triglyceride levels greater than 150 mg/dL.

PES4: Inadequate intake of vitamin D (NI-54.2) related to limited dietary intake as evidenced by nutrition assessment and serum 25(OH)D levels below 30 nd/mL.

Nutrition Intervention

With Carrie's parents present, the dietitian provided comprehensive nutrition education (E-2.0) regarding PCOS and insulin resistance and their connection with carbohydrate cravings and weight gain. The dietitian educated Carrie on the benefits of eating frequently throughout the day and including fiber-rich foods, protein, and fat with all meals and snacks to increase satiety and decrease carbohydrate cravings and hypoglycemia.

The benefits of listening to internal cues of hunger and satiety were discussed. Carrie agreed to keep food records, rating her hunger and satisfaction levels with meals.

Fish oil and vitamin D supplementation were recommended for elevated triglycerides and vitamin D deficiency. The benefits of physical activity were also discussed.

Dietary goals for Carrie focused on normalizing eating patterns and ending bingeing episodes and ultimately included the following:

- Record food intake, rating level of hunger
  and satisfaction with meals.
- Eat a midmorning snack.
- Include fiber-rich foods, protein, and fat at meals and snacks.
- Play Wii Sports three days per week for 30 minutes.
- Take 2,000 mg of fish oil daily.
- Take 5,000 IU of vitamin D daily.
- Schedule consultation with endocrinologist
  for further evaluation.

Monitoring and Evaluation

Carrie met with the dietitian twice a month for three months. Food records showed she increased her intake of whole grain carbohydrates and reduced her overall carbohydrate intake. She ate a midmorning snack at school and included protein and fat with her meals. She took nutrition supplements as prescribed.

Carrie rated her degree of hunger and fullness but was having difficulty distinguishing when she was satisfied. She noticed the connection between having more protein and fat with meals and reduced cravings for sweets, especially in the afternoon.

Carrie increased her activity level by playing Wii games three days per week, eventually finding a one-hour belly dancing class that she took two days per week.

Weekly follow-up sessions involved nutrition education on how food affects insulin levels. Food models were used to show Carrie serving sizes. Mindful eating exercises were used in nutrition sessions, which Carrie practiced at home to increase her knowledge of meal satisfaction. She saw an endocrinologist who prescribed 1,500 mg of metformin daily, which she tolerated well.

In three months, Carrie lost 5 lbs and was no longer bingeing, and her triglyceride and vitamin D levels were within normal levels.

CASE 3

Melissa was a 32-year-old woman referred for nutrition counseling by her doctor for PCOS, dyslipidemia, and hypertension. She had a family history of diabetes and hypertension. Her mother had diabetes, and Melissa didn't want to prick her fingers like her mother did.

She had been heavy since childhood. She had irregular menstrual periods and facial hair, and was obese.

Melissa's doctor had prescribed blood pressure medicine last year, but she had resisted taking it because she doesn't like to take pills. She was also prescribed metformin and lovaza, although she confessed that she took them sporadically.

Melissa was motivated to reduce her diabetes risk and stop taking medications. Melissa relied mostly on prepared foods, except for dinner, which her mother prepared. She said she's thirsty all the time and disliked water; she drank mostly sugary beverages.

She had a gym membership but never used it. Melissa's friend enjoyed aqua aerobics and had encouraged Melissa to join her, but Melissa didn't feel comfortable wearing a bathing suit in public. She did, however, enjoy dancing.

Recently, Melissa had become motivated to reduce her diabetes risk and stop taking medications.

Nutritional Assessment Data

1. Anthropometric Measurements
Height: 5'6"
Weight: 253 lbs
BMI: 41

2. Biochemical Data:

Parameter	Value	Normal Values (may vary by age, sex, and laboratory)
Total Testosterone	68	2-45 ng/dL
Glucose (fasting)	98	65-99 mg/dL
HbA1C	6.2	4.0 - 6.0%
Insulin (fasting)	18.4	2-20 uU/mL
TSH	1.63	40 – 5.50 uIU/mL
Total Cholesterol	263	<200 mg/dL

Continued on the next page

Parameter	Value	Normal Values (may vary by age, sex, and laboratory)
HDL Cholesterol	40	>46 mg/dL
LDL Cholesterol	183	<130 mg/dL
Triglycerides	530	<150 mg/dl

3. Nutrition-Focused Physical Findings

Patient has visible excess abdominal fat and facial hair.
Blood pressure: 142/91 mm Hg

4. Client History

The patient is 32 years old, works full-time as a receptionist, and
lives with her mother. The patient's mother and grandmother
have T2DM. She had limited cooking skills, relies on convenience
and fast foods during the day, and prepares only her evening meal
at home. She is inactive but has a gym membership.

5. Food/Nutrition-Related History

• Usual Diet

Breakfast (8:30 am)	Soft pretzel with mustard or muffin with butter, 16 oz juice
Snack (10 am)	Crackers, trail mix or a candy bar, 16 oz juice
Lunch (12 pm)	Hamburger or meatball sandwich, 16 oz soda, bag of chips or soup (chicken noodle)
Snack (2:30 pm)	Tea with sugar
Dinner (6:30 pm)	Beef, green beans, salad, two biscuits, 16 oz juice

• Medications: 2,000 mg metformin, 4 g lovaza, 50 mg carvedilol
• Supplements: None

Melissa did not drink alcohol, but she consumed 64 oz of fruit juice every day. She disliked water and artificial sweeteners. Breakfast consisted of highly refined carbohydrates and no protein. Lunch was fast food eaten during her break. Dinner was a homemade meal with several vegetables.

Her diet history showed Melissa ate a high amount of total calories, saturated fat, sodium, and refined carbohydrates. She generally did not consume antioxidant- and fiber-rich fruits and vegetables or calcium food sources. Most of her carbohydrate intake was from simple sugars, mostly from fruit juice and soda.

Nutrition Diagnosis

PES1: Excessive carbohydrate intake (NI-53.2) related to knowledge deficit as evidenced by diet history, consuming 64 oz of juice daily, fasting glucose of 104 mg/dL, and BMI of 41.

PES2: Excessive sodium intake (NI-55.2) related to diet intake as evidenced by blood pressure of 142/91 mm Hg and diet history.

PES3: Physical inactivity (NB-2.1) related to knowledge deficit as evidenced by no physical activity.

Nutrition Intervention

The dietitian provided nutrition counseling about the health risks associated with insulin resistance, hypertension, and excess body weight and how lifestyle changes could reduce these risks. Comprehensive nutrition education focused on how sugary beverages and excessive carbohydrate intake affect blood sugar.

Melissa stated her resistance to limiting her beverage intake. Motivational interviewing was used to encourage Melissa to decrease her intake of caloric beverages. Nutrition education about the sodium content of foods was discussed. The dietitian used food models and the plate method to educate Melissa on portion control. The health benefits of physical activity were also discussed.

With her new knowledge of her disease, Melissa was enthusiastic in making dietary changes to improve her PCOS symptoms and reduce her risk of diabetes.

Dietary and lifestyle goals for Melissa included a meal plan that supported a reduced calorie intake and achieving a 7% to 10%

reduction in body weight to improve glucose levels and decrease the risk of diabetes. More specifically, her goals were as follows:

- Limit the amount of fruit juice in her diet to 16 oz per day.
- Avoid high-sodium foods.
- Increase whole fruit consumption to one serving per day.
- Take prescribed medications daily.
- Keep food records.

Monitoring and Evaluation

Melissa consulted a dietitian because she wanted to reduce her risk of developing diabetes and stop taking her medications. Through intensive, personalized nutrition education and monitoring of her dietary and lifestyle changes at monthly follow-up appointments, the dietitian assisted Melissa in making changes in her diet to promote weight loss and improve insulin resistance, dyslipidemia, and blood pressure.

Continued follow-up sessions allowed the dietitian to work with Melissa on specific dietary goals that benefited her, such as the Dietary Approach to Stop Hypertension (DASH) diet for hypertension, increasing her intake of fiber-rich foods, and using a low-GI diet as a strategy to reduce insulin's response to carbohydrates.

Melissa and her dietitian worked on building lower-calorie and lower-sodium meal plans from restaurant menus. Melissa gradually reduced her intake of sugary beverages to 16 oz each day. She had been eating breakfast at home almost every day using the meal plans she created with the dietitian and ate a fresh fruit cup for her afternoon snack. She attended two ballroom dance classes each week and was enjoying them.

In three months, Melissa lost 8 lbs. New blood work showed slight reductions in fasting glucose, HbA1c, total cholesterol, and LDL cholesterol. Her triglyceride level was 430 mg/dL, and her blood pressure was 130/82—both significant reductions. Her overall caloric intake was reduced. She was now taking all her medications daily as directed, and her menstrual periods had regulated.

These case studies demonstrate the importance of MNT in the treatment of PCOS. Nutrition counseling regarding lifestyle modification is imperative since women with PCOS have a higher risk of developing chronic diseases, distorted eating, and infertility.

Lifestyle interventions for women with PCOS need to be individualized. Dietitians may find the use of food records, models, and labels helpful tools for providing nutrition counseling. Nutrition education and motivational interviewing can be used to facilitate behavior change. Adequate knowledge and training, along with a high degree of suspicion, can allow dietitians to identify patients who may have PCOS and recommend further diagnostic testing. Thus, dietitians play an important role in the recognition, prevention, and treatment of PCOS.

APPENDIX 1.
QUESTIONS TO ASK PATIENTS WITH SUSPECTED PCOS

"Tell me what your periods are like. Are they heavy, irregular, absent, etc.?"

"Do you struggle with acne anywhere on your body?"

"Do you ever feel lightheaded, dizzy, nauseous or irritable and do these get better when you eat?"

"Have you ever been told by your doctor or health care provider that you have any abnormal lab values (test results)?"

"Do you struggle with excessive facial or body hair?"

"What types of foods do you crave and when do you crave them?"

"Do you have dry/rough elbows or any dark patches that look dirty on your body?"

"Does anyone in your family have polycystic ovary syndrome?"

APPENDIX 2.
THE DIETITIAN'S TOOLBOX

The following are some helpful tools dietitians may want to use in providing medical nutrition therapy with their PCOS clients:

Food Models
The use of food models is a very effective way to educate clients on serving sizes of food. By actually viewing the portion size of a food, clients can better plan their meals and follow a meal plan (if they're on one). It is also very helpful for someone who eats out often to see what constitutes a serving. Food models can also be a valuable tool when discussing carbohydrate counting.

Label Reading

Reading food labels can be an effective way to educate patients on serving sizes of food and identify amounts of carbohydrate, fiber, sugar, sodium, fat and protein. Examining the ingredient list can show patients how to identify if a food is whole grain and what ingredients are in a food item. Clients' increased understanding of what to look for in a food item may assist them in selecting and preparing healthier foods.

Food Journaling

Although clients may dislike them (probably associated from negative past experiences with dieting), food journaling with the use of food records can be a very powerful tool for both clients and dietitians. Keeping a daily account of food eaten can give the dietitian a better idea of clients' food preferences and eating habits and can be used to monitor progress with changes in eating. It also helps clients become more self-aware and accountable of their own eating habits. Food journaling can assist clients who are trying to connect to their levels of hunger and satisfaction before and after meals. For clients who describe their mood and feelings associated with eating, food journaling can help overcome distorted eating by the use of reality checks and uncover connections between food and feelings.

The Scale

The scale is one tool used to measure clients' weight and may reflect changes (positive or negative) in eating, lifestyle and medication use. However, weight loss can be very slow for some women with PCOS and weight fluctuations are common. It is not unusual for women with PCOS to lose inches in body fat and not lose weight because they tend to gain muscle easily. For those that are exercising regularly, anthropometric measurements, such as waist circumference measurements, may be a more reliable tool.

Waist Circumference

Waist circumference (WC) independently predicts disease risk. Monitoring changes in WC over time (ideally monthly), may be helpful since it can provide an estimate of increased abdominal fat even without changes in BMI or weight. In women with PCOS who have metabolic complications, reductions in WC represent positive changes in CVD risk factors. WC is measured with the patient standing, at a point midway between the lower costal margin and iliac crest in the mid-axillary line. The waist circumference at which there is an increased relative disease risk in women is defined as >88 cm (>35 in).

1. Lemieux S, Prud'homme D, Bouchard C, Tremblay A, Despres JP. A single threshold value of waist girth identifies normal-weight and overweight subjects with excess visceral adipose tissue. Amer. j. clin. nutr. Nov 1996;64(5):685-693.
2. NHLBI Guidelines on Overweight and Obesity: Electronic Textbook accessed on April 14, 2013.http://www.nhlbi.nih.gov/guidelines/obesity/e_txtbk/txgd/4142.htm.

APPENDIX 3. SAMPLE MENU PLANS FOR PCOS

1200-1400 Calorie Sample Menu

Breakfast
1 cup blueberries
1 cup almond milk
¾ cup oatmeal, cooked
2 TBS slivered almonds

Lunch
4 oz shrimp
2 cups spinach salad with egg and mushrooms
Orange
8 walnuts
2 TBS Asian vinaigrette dressing

Snack
1 TBS almond butter
Apple
Dinner
5 oz pork tenderloin
1 cup mixed vegetables, steamed
1 tsp olive oil
¾ cup bulgur pilaf

27% protein, 40% carbohydrate, 33 g fiber, 45% fat,
5% saturated fat, 19% MUFA, 17% PUFA, 1919 mg sodium

1500-1700 Calorie Sample Menu

Breakfast
1 clementine
Egg sandwich with 1 egg, 1 slice of low fat cheese,
1 whole grain English muffin, 1 tsp butter

Snack
Small banana
1 TBS peanut butter

Lunch
3 oz turkey burger on whole grain roll
with lettuce, tomato, onion, ¼ avocado, mustard
1 cup baby carrots with 2 TBS hummus

Snack
10 cashews
½ cup fresh pitted cherries

Dinner
5 oz Grilled Salmon
1 tsp olive oil and 1 lemon
1 small sweet potato
Tomato Caprese salad: 1 oz fresh mozzarella cheese,
1 sliced tomato, 1 cup fresh arugula, 1 TBS olive oil,
fresh basil, 1TBS balsamic vinegar

25% protein, 35% carbohydrate, 28 g fiber, 40% fat, 9% saturated,
19% MUFA, 8% PUFA, 2,043 mg sodium

1800-2000 Calorie Sample Menu

Breakfast
Yogurt parfait: 6 oz low fat Greek yogurt with 1 cup raspberries,
¼ cup low sugar granola, 8 walnut halves

Snack
Green Smoothie (combine in blender):
1 green apple
1 cup almond milk
1 celery stalk
1½ cup kale

Lunch
1 whole grain pita
Greek Salad: 3 oz grilled, skinless chicken, 1 oz low fat feta cheese,
1½ cups mixed greens, 4 olives, 4 grape tomatoes, cucumber slices,
and slices of red onion with 1 TBS red wine vinaigrette
1 cup blueberries

Snack
3 cups popcorn, plain
1 cup coconut milk

Dinner
2 Fish Tacos on 6 inch whole wheat flour tortillas with
5 oz tuna steak, 2 TBS guacamole, 2 TBS fresh tomato salsa,
and ¼ cup shredded cabbage
½ cup black beans

27% protein, 49% carbohydrate, 38 g fiber, 27% fat, 6% saturated,
10% MUFA, 8% PUFA, 2,242 mg sodium

2000-2200 Calorie Sample Menu

Breakfast
2 egg omelet with 1 oz low-fat cheese, 2 slices whole grain bread,
1 cup mixed onions and peppers prepared with 2 tsp olive oil
1 cup strawberries

Snack
6 oz plain yogurt, nonfat
1 cup blueberries

Lunch
1 cup low sodium lentil soup
Chicken Caesar salad with 4 oz chicken,
2 cups kale, 2 TBS lite Caesar dressing

Snack
Banana Smoothie (combine in a blender):
1 TBS almond butter
1 cup almond milk
Small banana

Dinner
6 oz grilled halibut topped with 1 TBS pesto
1 cup quinoa mixed with ¼ cup yellow and orange peppers,
4 walnut halves and 1 TBS lite raspberry vinaigrette dressing
1 cup green beans
1.5 oz dark chocolate

21% protein, 46% carbohydrate, 45 g fiber, 35% fat, 8% saturated,
15% MUFA, 9% PUFA, 2,320 mg sodium

APPENDIX 4. PCOS RESOURCES

Androgen Excess and PCOS Society
www.ae-society.org
The Androgen Excess and PCOS Society is an international organization dedicated to promoting knowledge, and original clinical and basic research, in every aspect of androgen excess disorders. The Society disseminates information to the medical and scientific community, and the public. Member benefits include quarterly literature review, publications and annual conference.

Children's Hospital of Boston's Center for Young Women's Health
www.youngwomenshealth.org/pcosinfo.html
This site focuses on PCOS information for teens and has a great explanation of many common PCOS questions. It also includes tips on reading food labels, recipes, snack ideas, sample menus, and worksheets for menu planning and exercise, all specifically for the teen with PCOS.

Jean Hailes Managing PCOS
www.managingpcos.org.au
This website of an Australian Women's clinic, provides practical advice on diagnosis and management of PCOS, based on the latest research, for women and health professionals. Use this site to read PCOS evidence-based guidelines from the PCOS Australian Alliance.

PCOS Nutrition Center
www.PCOSnutrition.com
Founded by Angela Grassi, MS, RD, LDN author of *PCOS: The Dietitian's Guide* and *The PCOS Workbook: Your Guide to Complete Physical and Emotional Health*, the PCOS Nutrition Center provides reliable and objective nutrition information for PCOS. Sign up for the free monthly PCOS Nutrition Tips Newsletter and the PCOS Nutrition Center Blog. Nutrition counseling by phone, online, or in person for women with PCOS available.

PCOS Challenge
www.pcoschallenge.com
PCOS Challenge, is one of the largest and most active nonprofit support organizations for women with PCOS. In addition to their large message board, support groups, education and awareness initiatives, they offer recorded radio interviews with professionals who treat PCOS.

PCOS Guidebook for Teens
www.sites.google.com/site/teenpcosguidebook/
This site provides access to a beautifully illustrated and informational booklet designed to help teens better understand PCOS. Professionals can order copies of *The PCOS Guidebook* for patients and view it online.

PCOS Foundation
www.pcosfoundation.org
The mission of the PCOS Foundation is to spread awareness through public and professional education programs in order to improve diagnosis and decrease or eliminate the lifetime risks associated with PCOS. It offers support groups, a 5K run and other fundraising opportunities.

Polycystic Ovary Association
www.PCOSupport.org
The Polycystic Ovary Association is a grass-roots, volunteer-based organization, operated by and for women with PCOS. This website offers general information about PCOS and provides a message board.

Polycystic Ovary Syndrome of Australia
www.posaa.asn.au
This organization provides support, information, and advocacy for PCOS. The Australian website also includes chat rooms, message boards, professional database and annual conference.

Verity
www.verity-pcos.org.uk
Verity is the support organization for women with PCOS living in the United Kingdom. It provides a newsletter, discussion board, fact sheets and support groups. This organization also has an annual conference.

PCOS UK
www.pcos-uk.org.uk
PCOS UK provides educational support and resources for health care professionals caring for women with PCOS.

Soulcysters
www.soulcysters.com
A great resource for women with PCOS. This website provides a good overview of symptoms, treatment, and other PCOS links. Vast message board where individuals can post questions and read others responses on different topics related to PCOS.

American Society for Reproductive Medicine
www.asrm.org
The ASRM, which has a nutrition subgroup, is a multidisciplinary organization committed to the advancement of reproductive medicine by serving as the leading advocate for patient care, research and education. ASRM has information on infertility for professionals and consumers. Use the website to find a doctor. Provides annual conference.

National Eating Disorders Association
www.edap.org
A great resource that provides information and advocacy for eating disorders. Use this site to locate a treatment professional or download reproducible fact sheets and client handouts. This organization hosts an annual conference for consumers and professionals.

RESOLVE: The National Infertility Association
www.resolve.org
RESOLVE is a non-profit organization to promote reproductive health and to ensure equal access to all family building options for men and women experiencing infertility or other reproductive disorders. Resolve provides awareness, support and information to people who are experiencing infertility.

APPENDIX 5.
COMMON IDC-10 CODES FOR PCOS
AND RELATED CONDITIONS

IDC-9 Code	IDC-10 Code	Diagnosis
706.10	L70.90	Acne, unspecified
704.00	L65.90	Alopecia
626.00	N91.0	Amenorrhea
307.10	F50.0	Anorexia nervosa
307.51	F50.2	Bulimia nervosa
250.00	E11.0	Diabetes types 2
579.00	K90.0	Celiac disease
307.50	F50.9	Eating disorder not otherwise specified
648.83	Z86.32	Gestational diabetes mellitus
271.90	R73.02	Impaired glucose tolerance
704.10	L68.0	Hirsutism
272.00	E78.0	Hypercholesterolemia
401.10	I15.2	Hypertension

IDC-9 Code	IDC-10 Code	Diagnosis
790.60	R73.9	Hyperglycemia (without diabetes)
272.20	E78.5	Hyperlipidemia, mixed
251.10	E16.1	Hyperinsulinism
272.10	E78.1	Hypertriglyceridemia
251.20	E16.2	Hypoglycemia, unspecified, nondiabetic
244.90	E03.9	Hypothyroidism
628.90	N97.9	Infertility, unspecified
564.10	K58.9	Irritable bowel syndrome
277.70	E88.81	Metabolic syndrome
278.00	E66.9	Obesity, NOS (not otherwise specified)
733.90	M85.80	Osteopenia
733.00	Q78.2	Osteoporosis
278.02	E66.3	Overweight
256.40	E28.2	Polycycstic ovary syndrome
642.40	O14.00	Preeclampsia
327.23	G47.3	Obstructive sleep apnea

INDEX

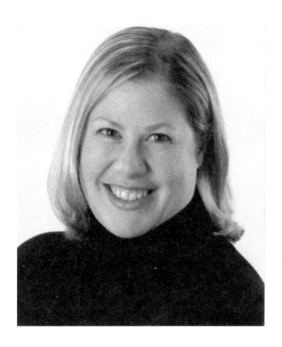

ABOUT THE AUTHOR

Angela Grassi, MS, RD, LDN is the author of *PCOS: The Dietitian's Guide,* and is co-author of *The PCOS Workbook: Your Guide to Complete Physical and Emotional Health.* She also wrote the PCOS chapter in The Academy of Nutrition and Dietetics *Nutrition Care Manual.* In 2013, Angela received The Award for Excellence in Women's Health and is a past recipient of The Award for Excellence in Graduate Research, both from the Academy of Nutrition and Dietetics. Angela is the founder of the PCOS Nutrition Center where she provides evidence-based nutrition information and nutrition counseling to women with PCOS around the world. She speaks frequently to consumers and professionals. Having PCOS herself, Angela has been dedicated to advocacy, education, and research of the syndrome. She resides in the Philadelphia area with her husband and two sons. For more information or to sign up for her PCOS Nutrition Tips Newsletter visit her website, www.PCOSnutrition.com.

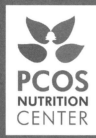
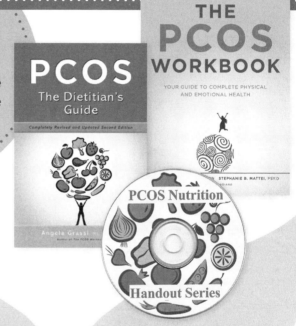